BROCKPORT PHYSICAL FITNESS TEST MANUAL

A Health-Related Assessment for Youngsters With Disabilities

Second Edition

Joseph P. Winnick

Francis X. Short

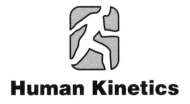

Human Kinetics

Library of Congress Cataloging-in-Publication Data

Winnick, Joseph P., author.
  Brockport physical fitness test manual : a health-related assessment for youngsters with disabilities / Joseph P. Winnick and Francis X. Short. -- Second edition.
       pages cm
  Includes bibliographical references and index.
  ISBN-13: 978-1-4504-6869-5 (print)
  ISBN-10: 1-4504-6869-1 (print)
  1. Physical fitness for children--Testing--Handbooks, manuals, etc. 2. Exercise therapy for children--Handbooks, manuals, etc. 3. Children with disabilities--Development--Handbooks, manuals, etc. I. Short, Francis X. (Francis Xavier), 1950- author. II. Title.
  RJ138.W55 2014
  613.7'042087--dc23
                          2014002585

ISBN-10: 1-4504-6869-1 (print)
ISBN-13: 978-1-4504-6869-5 (print)

Acquisitions Editor: Scott Wikgren; **Developmental Editor:** Ragen E. Sanner; **Associate Managing Editor:** B. Rego; **Assistant Editor:** Anne Rumery; **Copyeditor:** Tom Tiller; **Indexer:** Bobbi Swanson; **Permissions Manager:** Dalene Reeder; **Graphic Designer:** Joe Buck; **Graphic Artist:** Kathleen Boudreau-Fuoss; **Cover Designer:** Keith Blomberg; **Photographs (interior):** © Human Kinetics, unless otherwise noted; figures 5.5, 5.15, and 5.30 courtesy of Matthew J. Yeoman; **Photo Asset Manager:** Laura Fitch; **Visual Production Assistant:** Joyce Brumfield; **Photo Production Manager:** Jason Allen; **Art Manager:** Kelly Hendren; **Associate Art Manager:** Alan L. Wilborn; **Illustrations:** © Human Kinetics; **Printer:** Sheridan Books

The video contents of this product are licensed for educational public performance for viewing by a traditional (live) audience, via closed circuit television, or via computerized local area networks within a single building or geographically unified campus. To request a license to broadcast these contents to a wider audience—for example, throughout a school district or state, or on a television station—please contact your sales representative (**www.HumanKinetics.com/SalesRepresentatives**).

Printed in the United States of America   10 9 8 7 6 5 4 3 2 1

The paper in this book is certified under a sustainable forestry program.

Human Kinetics
Website: www.HumanKinetics.com

United States: Human Kinetics
P.O. Box 5076
Champaign, IL 61825-5076
800-747-4457
e-mail: humank@hkusa.com

Canada: Human Kinetics
475 Devonshire Road Unit 100
Windsor, ON N8Y 2L5
800-465-7301 (in Canada only)
e-mail: info@hkcanada.com

Europe: Human Kinetics
107 Bradford Road
Stanningley
Leeds LS28 6AT, United Kingdom
+44 (0) 113 255 5665
e-mail: hk@hkeurope.com

Australia: Human Kinetics
57A Price Avenue
Lower Mitcham, South Australia 5062
08 8372 0999
e-mail: info@hkaustralia.com

New Zealand: Human Kinetics
P.O. Box 80
Torrens Park, South Australia 5062
0800 222 062
e-mail: info@hknewzealand.com

Contents

Preface   v

Use of the Term *Healthy Fitness Zone*®   vii

Acknowledgments   ix

How to Use the Web Resource   xi

1 Introduction to the Brockport Physical Fitness Test 1

2 The Conceptual Framework 7

3 Using the Brockport Physical Fitness Test 23

4 Profiles, Test Selection Guides, Standards, and Fitness Zones 29

5 Test Administration and Test Items 55

6 Testing Youngsters With Severe Disability 101

Appendix A   Body Mass Index (BMI) Chart   105

Appendix B   Purchasing and Constructing Unique Testing Supplies   107

Appendix C   Fitnessgram Body Composition Conversion Charts   115

Appendix D   PACER Conversion Chart   117

Appendix E   Data Forms   119

Appendix F   Frequently Asked Questions   125

Appendix G   Teacher and Parent Overview   129

Glossary   131

References and Resources   133

Index   135

Contributors   143

About the Authors   147

Preface

In 1993, the U.S. Department of Education funded Project Target, a research study designed primarily to develop a health-related, criterion-referenced physical fitness test for youngsters aged 10 to 17 with disability. Project Target was centered at the College at Brockport, State University of New York; it was directed by Joseph P. Winnick and coordinated by Francis X. Short. Two important goals of the project were to develop standards for attaining healthful living through physical fitness and to help young people with disability develop health-related fitness.

The test developed through Project Target has been designated as the Brockport Physical Fitness Test (BPFT). It was first published in 1999, then revised in 2014. This manual presents information necessary to understand the test, administer test items, and interpret the results. Detailed information about the test's validity and reliability can be found in Winnick and Short (2005).

The first chapter of this manual introduces the test and identifies, defines, and classifies its target populations. This information is critical for all testers because test item selection and criterion-referenced standards are tied to classifications and subclassifications of disability.

The second chapter presents the test's conceptual framework. Specifically, it discusses physical activity, health, and health-related physical fitness, as well as their interrelationships for the purposes of the BPFT. It also describes a personalized approach to physical fitness testing, which includes the following elements: identifying health-related concerns, creating a desired physical fitness profile that emerges from the identified health-related concerns, selecting the components of physical fitness to be measured, identifying test items that measure the selected components, and selecting and applying health-related standards and fitness zones in order to assess physical fitness.

Chapter 3 presents three options for using the BPFT: (1) using only BPFT test items and standards, (2) adjusting the BPFT for youngsters with disability, and (3) combining the BPFT with tests used for youngsters without disability or with other disability-specific tests. The final section of this chapter briefly addresses development of an individualized education program (IEP).

The fourth chapter presents health-related, criterion-referenced test selection guides, standards, and fitness zones for assessing physical fitness. This information is presented in tables that identify health-related parameters both for young people in the general population and for those with specific disabilities.

Chapter 5 includes general recommendations for test administration and specific instructions for administering test items. All 27 BPFT test items are presented, though the number of items administered to each individual generally ranges from four to six. The chapter also discusses test item objectives, how to administer the items, what equipment is needed, ways of scoring, trials required, and test modifications. Test items are presented within categories that reflect the components of physical fitness used in the study: aerobic functioning, body composition, and musculoskeletal functioning (including muscular strength and endurance, as well as flexibility or range of motion).

The sixth chapter covers the testing of physical fitness in youngsters with severe disability. During the BPFT design process, it became obvious that a single physical fitness test could not accommodate all disabilities or levels of function. The BPFT is appropriate for most youngsters with disability and unique physical fitness needs; however, it may not be appropriate for those with severe disability. This chapter offers two orientations for measuring physical fitness or physical activity in individuals with severe disability—one related to alternative assessment and the other related to the measurement of physical activity.

This manual also includes several appendixes to support test implementation and further inform consumers. Appendix A provides a convenient, user-friendly reference for determining body mass index. Appendix B provides information about purchasing and constructing unique testing supplies. Appendix C enables users to quickly determine (without computer assistance) percent body fat for males and females from the sum of triceps and calf skinfolds. Appendix D enables users to easily convert PACER 15-meter lap scores to 20-meter lap scores. Appendix E provides two sample forms for collecting and interpreting data using the BPFT; these forms can help determine data needed for analysis and how to record data for interpretation. Appendixes F and G answer frequently asked questions about the BPFT, discuss the basis for the test, and provide help for interpreting test results. In addition, the manual includes a glossary of terms and a list of the many contributors to the project.

This edition of the BPFT manual also includes an accompanying web resource, which offers video clips, reproducible forms, and informational fitness zone charts. The web resource can be found at www.HumanKinetics.com/BrockportPhysical FitnessTestManual and can be accessed by using the pass code Brockport58743AR7. The reproducible items can be printed from the web resource for easy use within the classroom. For more information, please see the section titled How to Use the Web Resource in this manual.

In presenting the BPFT, we wish to emphasize that we consider the assessment of health-related physical fitness in youngsters with disability to be a work in progress. There is little question that the test items, standards, and fitness zones suggested in this manual will require continued scrutiny and study. We encourage further research in this field.

Use of the Term *Healthy Fitness Zone*®

We use the term *Healthy Fitness Zone (HFZ)* to refer both to general standards that were developed by the Cooper Institute (Dallas, Texas) specifically for the Fitnessgram test and to general standards developed in Project Target that were created specifically for the Brockport Physical Fitness Test. The term *Healthy Fitness Zone* is a registered trademark of the Cooper Institute. It is used in this manual by permission of the Cooper Institute for the purpose of giving youth with disability and their parents and guardians a report that is understandable and consistent with the reports received by all students using Fitnessgram.

We and the Cooper Institute strongly advocate that all students have access to high-quality physical education and appropriate health-related fitness assessment. We appreciate the Cooper Institute's willingness to help us create consistent reports for youngsters with disability that allow them to participate, to the extent possible, in Fitnessgram and to have those scores included with the Brockport Physical Fitness Test scores so that just one report is necessary.

The connection between Fitnessgram and the Brockport Physical Fitness Test is further evidenced by the adoption of both by the Presidential Youth Fitness Program. For more information about that program, go to www.pyfp.org.

Trademark *Healthy Fitness Zone* (HFZ)® is used by permission of The Cooper Institute.

Acknowledgments

The Brockport Physical Fitness Test (BPFT) was initially developed with the help of a diverse group of people and institutions as part of Project Target. The project could not have been completed without the cooperation of many individuals, schools, and agencies throughout the United States. Nor did the project have the resources to fully compensate individuals for their contributions. Those who helped did so in the belief that the resulting project would enhance the health-related fitness of individuals with disabilities. The names of individuals and educational institutions that made contributions to the project appear at the end of this manual. We extend deep gratitude to these people and organizations. Our thanks are also given to the many parents and youngsters who volunteered their time and effort for testing purposes. They also believed that the project would bring benefits to young people with disability.

Some individuals made extraordinary contributions to this project. At the forefront of these contributors was the Project Target Advisory Committee. The members of the advisory board provided guidance to Project Target in general and to the development of this test manual in particular. They also served as a panel of experts in the development of criterion-referenced standards. The original advisory committee members and their associations during their contributions were Kirk J. Cureton, PhD, University of Georgia; Harold W. Kohl, PhD, Baylor Sports Medicine Institute; Kenneth Richter, DO, medical director, United States Cerebral Palsy Athletic Association; James H. Rimmer, PhD, Northern Illinois University; Margaret Jo Safrit, PhD, American University; Roy J. Shephard, MD, PhD, DPE, University of Toronto (retired); and Julian U. Stein, EdD, George Mason University (retired).

Paul Surburg at Indiana University deserves special recognition. Paul gave continued advice about the development of test items and standards associated with flexibility and range of motion. Special recognition is also extended to Bo Fernhall at George Washington University. Bo gave the project much insight in the area of aerobic fitness for individuals with disability and conducted valuable research for the development of the BPFT. Patrick DiRocco of the University of Wisconsin at La Crosse gave valuable input on test items related to musculoskeletal functioning.

Special appreciation goes to Pam Maryjanowski, who was associated with the Empire State Games for the Physically Challenged. Pam was particularly helpful in gaining access to subjects for the study. Two other individuals who also made the project's data collection possible were Paul Ponchillia, Western Michigan University, and Sister Seraphine Herbst, director of the School of the Holy Childhood in Rochester, New York. Arnie Epstein and Bob Lewis from the New York City Public Schools were extremely helpful in organizing data collection efforts in that school district. Each of these people very willingly and ably contributed to data collection efforts that were important for the development of the BPFT.

One important function in the development of standards for the BPFT was to test a general population of youngsters (i.e., those without disability). The Brockport Central School District was very important in this regard. More than 900 students were tested in the district, and the resulting data served as a source for the development of health-related, criterion-referenced physical fitness standards. Thanks are given to the administrators of the school district and to the 15 physical education teachers associated with the district who cooperated and gave much help when their students were tested. Finally, thanks to Joe Setek from Brockport Central for his contributions to the video activities in this project.

Gratitude is expressed to Richard Incardona for helping prepare the art. Thanks also are given to students who posed for pictures or sketches in the 1999 manual, including Kevin Wexler, Kelda DePrez, Lori Volding, Travis Phillips, Tucker Short, and Stephanie White. Several young people with disability also posed for pictures. In 2013, video resources for the BPFT were revised. Thanks are particularly expressed to subjects and their devoted parents for their help in this endeavor. Gratitude is also given to Brockport students for demonstrating the teaching of test items in video resources. These include Caitlyn Rana, Tom Rispoli, Gabriella Badalucco, Tiffany Mitrakos, Jorge Baez, Anthony Miller, and Timothy Bush. Jack Hogan and Octavio Furtado graciously provided needed logistical and administrative support throughout the process. Appreciation also is extended to Pam Turner, who provided secretarial support for this second edition.

Thanks are extended to the professional organizations that endorsed and cooperated with the original project. The American Alliance for Health, Physical Education, Recreation and Dance (AAHPERD) and the National Consortium for Physical Education and Recreation for Individuals with Disabilities (NCPERID) supported the original proposal for funding the project and provided opportunities for several presentations regarding the BPFT at professional meetings. Gratitude is also extended to the Cooper Institute in Dallas, Texas. Their work with Fitnessgram served as a prototype for the BPFT, and several test items and standards from Fitnessgram are used by the BPFT, thus enhancing the link between the two tests.

How to Use the Web Resource

This second edition of the *Brockport Physical Fitness Test Manual* includes access to a web resource that will help administer the test. Visit the web resource at www.HumanKinetics. com/BrockportPhysicalFitnessTestManual and sign in using the pass code Brockport58743AR7 to access the accompanying video clips, fitness zone charts, and reproducible forms.

Video

The Brockport Physical Fitness Test (BPFT) video materials include segments introducing and overviewing the test. Specifically, they present background information about the meaning and benefits of health-related physical fitness; the theoretical basis and constructs underlying the BPFT; the nature of health-related, criterion-referenced assessment; components of health-related physical fitness; and test items included in the BPFT. They also briefly describe the target populations with disability, including classifications and subclassifications associated with particular disabilities, and offer guidelines for selecting test items.

In addition, the video materials present steps for developing a personalized physical fitness test based on an individual's health-related needs. They also discuss the basis for evaluating fitness via specific and general standards and how they apply to interpreting results, with emphasis on three levels of fitness: needs improvement, adapted fitness zone, and Healthy Fitness Zone.

Most of the remaining video materials are devoted to demonstrating the BPFT test items themselves. For each item, the materials cover the purpose, procedures, number of test trials, scoring instructions, and any special considerations. They also summarize guidelines for a safe and effective assessment experience.

The icon shown in figure 1 appears with the test descriptions in chapter 5 as a reminder that video samples are available.

Figure 1 The video icon appears at key points in the text of the manual to point toward the accompanying video material.

Reproducible Materials

The web resource includes a variety of reproducible materials designed to help users, particularly school teachers, enhance and simplify their data collection and reporting and disseminate reports and other information to participants, parents, schools, and other constituencies. Examples of possible uses include bulletin boards, individual report cards, and class and school summary reports. Available items include a physical fitness profile sheet, fitness zone tables, the target stretch test, and two forms for collecting and interpreting individual data using the BPFT.

The icon shown in figure 2 appears in the manual with forms and other materials available for printing in the web resource.

Figure 2 The reproducibles icon appears with materials in the book that are also available for printing from the web resource.

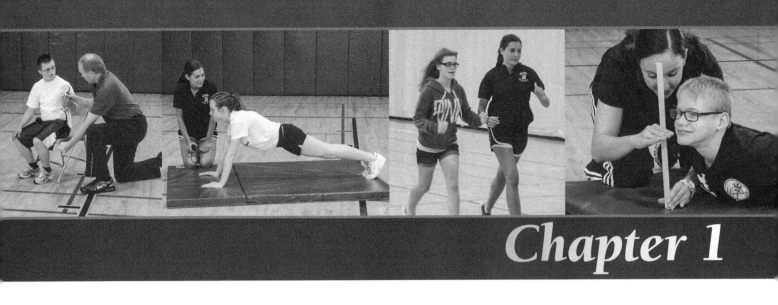

Chapter 1

Introduction to the Brockport Physical Fitness Test

The Brockport Physical Fitness Test (BPFT) is a health-related, criterion-referenced test of fitness. The term *health-related* is used to distinguish objectives of this test battery from others that might be more appropriately related to skill or physical performance. The phrase *criterion-referenced* conveys that the standards for evaluation are based on values believed to have significance for an individual's health. **Criterion-referenced standards** can be established in a number of ways, including through research findings, logic, expert opinion, and norm-referenced data (e.g., averages, percentiles).

The BPFT is designed primarily for use among youngsters with disability. It is particularly compatible with Fitnessgram®, the fitness test developed by the Cooper Institute® (2013).

In the mid-1990s, the American Alliance for Health, Physical Education, Recreation and Dance (AAHPERD) adopted the Prudential Fitnessgram (Cooper Institute for Aerobics Research, 1992) as its recommended health-related, criterion-referenced test of **physical fitness**. However, while the Prudential Fitnessgram manual contained a section addressing special populations, different or modified test items and standards were not presented in a systematic way for young people with specific disabilities.

To address this need, the College at Brockport, State University of New York, received funding from the Office of Special Education and Rehabilitative Services in the U.S. Department of Education from 1993 to 1998 to support the work of Project Target (1998). The project aimed to develop a health-related, criterion-referenced physical fitness test for young people (aged 10 to 17) with disability. A key element of the project was to develop standards that would provide targets for attaining health-related physical fitness.

Another key goal of Project Target was to develop an educational component to enhance the development of health-related fitness in youngsters with disability. The populations targeted in this project included youth with mental retardation, spinal cord injury, cerebral palsy, blindness, congenital anomaly, or amputation. (In this current revision of the BPFT, the term *mental retardation* has been replaced by *intellectual disability* in order to be consistent with current conventions.)

Although the project targeted these particular disabilities, it also provides a process that can be used to assess the physical fitness of youngsters with other disabilities. During the project, a total of 1,542 young people (with and without disability) were tested, and data from several other projects (including thousands of youngsters) were also analyzed as part of Project Target. The result of Project Target is the Brockport Physical Fitness Test.

This second edition of the BPFT retains information about the test's background, definitions and classifications of disabilities, test items, test selection guides, and standards (slightly revised) for assessing performance. Some technical information from the first edition is not included here, but it can be found in Winnick and Short (2005). New and revised features of the second edition include a test manual with instructional video clips and reproducibles available in the accompanying web resource.

The BPFT includes a number of unique elements. First, it represents an initial attempt to apply a health-related, criterion-referenced fitness approach to youngsters with disability. Second, it recognizes the individualized nature of fitness testing and encourages a personalized approach based on health-related needs and a desired fitness **profile**. Third, in an effort to provide options for test administrators to personalize testing, the battery includes several test items from which to choose. Finally, some of the test items presented are new (or at least nontraditional) and are designed to include a larger number of individuals in the testing program than was previously possible.

This test manual is fairly thick. Many of the pages are dedicated to the directions for administering individual test items that are presented in chapter 5. Testers, however, should also become familiar with the material presented in other chapters because understanding the rationale for the test (along with its strengths and weaknesses) is important in interpreting results.

Test Construction

The BPFT includes 27 test items, but, generally speaking, only 4 to 6 items are needed in order to assess the health-related physical fitness of a particular individual. As expected, considerable study was undertaken to determine what test items to recommend in the test and what standards and fitness zones should be used to evaluate physical fitness. The process developed for

selecting test items and standards for youngsters reflects the **personalized approach** described in detail in chapter 2. The steps include identifying and selecting health-related concerns of importance for an individual, establishing a desired personalized fitness profile, selecting components and subcomponents of physical fitness to assess, selecting test items to measure the selected components, and selecting health-related standards and fitness zones to evaluate physical fitness.

In selecting test items and standards for the BPFT, one of the primary criteria used was validity. Once a conceptual framework was established for health-related physical fitness, test items and standards were selected on the basis of logic, literature review, and data deemed relevant to validity. The theoretical conceptual basis for the test's validity is more specifically discussed and summarized in Winnick and Short (2005).

A second criterion for selection of test items was reliability. All of the test items recommended are believed to be reliable. Many data were found in the literature regarding the reliability of test items, and additional data supporting test-item reliability were collected as part of Project Target. Again, readers can obtain detailed information about the test's reliability in Winnick and Short (2005).

A third criterion for selection of test items and standards was the extent to which test items could be used for different categories of youngsters. Preference was given to test items and standards that could be applied to young people with and without disability and that could be found in appropriate tests of physical fitness designed for the general population. In particular, test items from Fitnessgram were selected so that the BPFT could be easily coordinated with that test. Preference was also given to test items that could be administered to both males and females, to youngsters between 10 and 17 years of age, and to young people with various disabilities.

The fourth criterion of primary importance was for test items to be suitable for measuring different physical fitness traits or abilities but also to encompass the components of physical fitness selected and defined for this test. This approach was taken so that each item in the test added new information about an individual's ability.

Additional secondary criteria were also applied in the selection of test items. Specifically, to the extent possible, preference was given to items reasonably familiar to physical educators, economical in terms of time and expense, and easily administered in field situations.

Target Populations

The BPFT was targeted for use among youngsters with disability—specifically, those with visual impairment, intellectual disability, or orthopedic impairment, including cerebral palsy, spinal cord injury, congenital anomaly, and amputation. However, it builds on and closely relates to physical fitness tests of youth in the general population, particularly Fitnessgram. Youngsters in the general population, of course, include those without disability (that is, those who are free from impairment or disability that influences test results).

The following sections present definitions and classifications associated with groups with whom the BPFT might be used.

Youngsters With Intellectual Disability

The first disability classification associated with this test is intellectual disability. Its definition is based on the American Association on Mental Retardation's (1992) definition of (in the terminology commonly used at the time) mental retardation:

> Mental retardation refers to substantial limitations in present functioning. It is characterized by significantly subaverage intellectual functioning, existing concurrently with related limitations in two or more of the following applicable adaptive skill areas: communication, self-care, home living, social skills, community use, self-direction, health and safety, functional academics, leisure, and work. Mental retardation manifests before age 18.

This definition includes three major criteria for the determination of an intellectual disability: subaverage intellectual functioning, deficits in adaptive behavior, and manifestation before age 18. This edition of the BPFT uses the term *intellectual disability* instead of *mental retardation*.

Although many youngsters with intellectual disability have no limitation in physical fitness, others exhibit limitations ranging from mild to severe. As a result, they may require slight to marked modifications in testing to measure physical fitness.

Youngsters with intellectual disability and mild limitations in physical fitness include both people who require intermittent or limited support in learning or performing test items and people who require substantial modification in test items or alternative test items to measure components of physical fitness. These individuals are capable of levels of fitness consistent with good health, can participate in games and leisure activities in selected appropriate environments, and can perform activities of daily living. Youngsters with intellectual disability and mild limitations are perhaps best associated with the lower levels of the "mild mental retardation" and "moderate mental retardation" classifications used in previous classification systems.

Youngsters with intellectual disability who have severe limitations generally need extensive or pervasive support related to physical fitness. These individuals require significant help in learning and performing physical fitness test items. They also need alternative test items or marked modification in measuring a component (or more than one) of physical fitness. As a result, valid assessment of physical fitness may not be possible in this group using typical health-related physical fitness tests. Thus, for this group, measurement of physical activity may be preferred over assessment that uses physical fitness test items.

Suitable test items of physical fitness for this group may include alternative assessments, such as rubrics and task-analyzed test items. In addition, these individuals often require physical assistance as they perform test items. (These approaches are discussed in greater detail in chapter 6.)

Table 1.1 summarizes limitations and needs related to physical fitness testing of youngsters with intellectual disability.

Youngsters With Visual Impairment

Visual impairment is defined as impairment in vision that, even with correction, adversely affects a child's educational performance. It includes both partial sight and blindness. Categories of blindness given in table 1.2 are consistent with those used by the U.S. Association of Blind Athletes (USABA). The partial-sight category used with this test corresponds to the B4 category developed by the USABA classification for sport competition.

Youngsters With Spinal Cord Injury

For purposes of the BPFT, a spinal cord injury is a condition that involves damage to the spinal cord resulting in motor and possibly sensory and muscular impairment. It includes traumatic as well as congenital spinal cord injury or malfunction. Both the level and the extent of damage affect the nature and degree of a person's impairment and disability. A complete spinal cord injury results in total loss of sensory, motor, and autonomic functions below the neurological level of spinal cord damage. An incomplete injury results in a partial but not total loss of function below the level of injury on the spinal cord.

The BPFT includes test items for individuals who have low-level quadriplegia or paraplegia and who primarily use wheelchairs for locomotion in their activities of daily living. These test items can also be used for ambulatory youngsters with spinal cord injury. To enable selection of appropriate test items and standards for measuring and evaluating physical fitness, the BPFT uses a three-category classification of spinal cord injury: low-level quadriplegia (LLQ), paraplegia—wheelchair (PW), and paraplegia—ambulatory (PA). See table 1.3 for more detail.

Youngsters With Cerebral Palsy

In order to group and categorize physical fitness test items and performance for this population, the BPFT has adopted the definition of cerebral palsy and the classification system used by the Cerebral Palsy International Sports and Recreation Association (CPISRA, 1993). Here is the definition:

Table 1.1 Limitations and Needs of Youngsters With Intellectual Disability in Physical Fitness Testing

Limitation	Needs
None	These individuals have no unique physical fitness needs and require no unique modification or support in learning and performing physical fitness tests. The desired physical fitness profile and standards for evaluating physical fitness are identical to those for youngsters without disability.
Mild	These individuals have mild limitations in physical fitness requiring intermittent or limited support in learning or performing test items. They may also require substantial modification of test items or alternative test items to measure components of physical fitness. They can demonstrate physical fitness on an achievement scale. Adjusted standards for assessing physical fitness may be appropriate. The desired physical fitness profile leans toward or closely relates to that of youngsters without disability.
Severe	Because of severe limitations, these individuals need extensive or pervasive support in learning and performing test items. They also need alternative test items or marked modification in measuring components of physical fitness. They may require assessment involving physical activity rather than physical fitness. They generally need individualized criterion-referenced standards for assessment of physical fitness.

Table 1.2 Classification System for Youngsters With Visual Impairment

Category	Description
B1	Individuals who are totally blind (may possess light perception but are unable to recognize hand shapes at any distance)
B2	Individuals who can perceive hand shapes but with visual acuity of not better than 20/600 or who have less than 5° in the visual field
B3	Individuals with visual acuity from 20/599 to 20/200 and those with 5° through 20° in the visual field
PS	Individuals who are partially sighted (those with visual acuity from 20/199 to 20/70)

Cerebral palsy is a brain lesion which is nonprogressive and causes variable impairment of the coordination, tone and strength of muscle action with resulting inability of the person to maintain normal postures and perform normal movements.

In order to describe degree of impairment as it influences performance in physical activity and sport, this test has adapted and collected test data for a classification system originally developed by CPISRA (1993) based on a functional evaluation that includes assessing the extent of an individual's control of the lower extremity, trunk, upper extremity, and hand. This classification system is summarized in table 1.4.

Category C1 includes individuals with the most severe involvement (e.g., those who depend on an electric wheelchair or assistance for mobility),

Table 1.3 Classification System for Youngsters With Spinal Cord Injury

Category	Description
Low-level quadriplegia (LLQ)	Individuals with complete or incomplete spinal cord damage that results in neurological impairment of all four extremities and the trunk, as well as individuals with lower cervical (C6–C8) neurological involvement
Paraplegia—wheelchair (PW)	Individuals with complete or incomplete spinal cord injury below the cervical area resulting in motor loss in the lower extremities (paraplegia) and the need to use a wheelchair for daily living activities
Paraplegia—ambulatory (PA)	Individuals with complete or incomplete spinal cord injury resulting in motor loss in the lower extremities but who ambulate in daily activities without wheelchair assistance

Table 1.4 Classification System for Youngsters With Cerebral Palsy

Category	Description
C1	Individuals with severe spastic quadriplegia, with or without athetosis, or with poor functional range of movement and poor functional strength in all extremities and trunk; and individuals with severe athetoid quadriplegia, with or without spasticity, with poor functional strength and control. In either case, these individuals depend on an electric wheelchair or assistance for mobility and are unable to functionally propel a manual wheelchair.
C2	Individuals with severe to moderate spastic quadriplegia, with or without athetosis, or with severe athetoid quadriplegia with fair function in the less-affected side. These individuals have poor functional strength in all extremities and trunk but are able to propel a manual wheelchair. Further classifications are C2U if the individual exhibits relatively better upper-body abilities than lower-body abilities and C2L if the individual exhibits relatively greater lower-body than upper-body abilities.
C3	Individuals with moderate quadriplegia or severe hemiplegia resulting in use of a wheelchair for activities of daily living who can propel a manual wheelchair independently and have almost full functional strength in the dominant upper extremity.
C4	Individuals with moderate to severe diplegia with good functional strength and minimal limitation or control problems in the upper limbs or trunk. A wheelchair is usually chosen for sport.
C5	Individuals with moderate diplegia or triplegia who may require the use of assistive devices in walking but not necessarily when standing or throwing. Problems with dynamic balance are possible.
C6	Individuals with moderate athetosis or ataxia who ambulate without aids. Athetosis is the most prevalent factor, although some individuals with spastic quadriplegia (i.e., more arm involvement than in ambulant diplegia) may fit this classification. All four limbs usually show functional involvement in sport movements. Individuals in the C6 class usually have more control problems in upper limbs than those in C5 but usually have better function in lower limbs, particularly when running.
C7	Individuals with ambulant hemiplegia and spasticity on one side of the body who ambulate without an assistive device but often with a limp due to spasticity in a lower limb. These individuals have good functional ability on the dominant side of the body.
C8	Individuals who are minimally affected by spastic diplegia, spastic hemiplegia, or monoplegia or who are minimally affected by athetosis or ataxia.

Adapted, by permission, from Cerebral Palsy International Sport and Recreation Association (CP-ISRA), 1993, *CP-ISRA handbook*, 5th ed. (Heteren, Netherlands: CP-ISRA).

Readers interested in subsequent changes made in this classification system should consult the Blaze Sports (www.blazesports.org).

whereas category C8, the highest class, includes those who are minimally affected (e.g., those who can run and jump freely). The first four classes are appropriate for individuals who use wheelchairs, and the second four are appropriate for those who are ambulatory. Although the system has been modified by Blaze Sports America, the 1993 system is used with the BPFT so as to be consistent with data collected during Project Target.

Youngsters With Congenital Anomaly or Amputation

For the purposes of the BPFT, individuals with congenital anomaly include youngsters with fully or partially deformed extremities at birth, whereas individuals with amputation are missing part or all of an extremity (or more than one). Amputation may be congenital or acquired. The BPFT's classification system, tests, and standards assume that these individuals are nondisabled except for their congenital anomaly or amputation. Individuals who have physical conditions or diseases in addition to congenital anomaly or amputation must have programs more specifically personalized for them with medical consultation.

For the BPFT, individuals are subclassified according to limb involvement. The specific location of limb involvement (right or left side) is not typically a factor in subclassification.

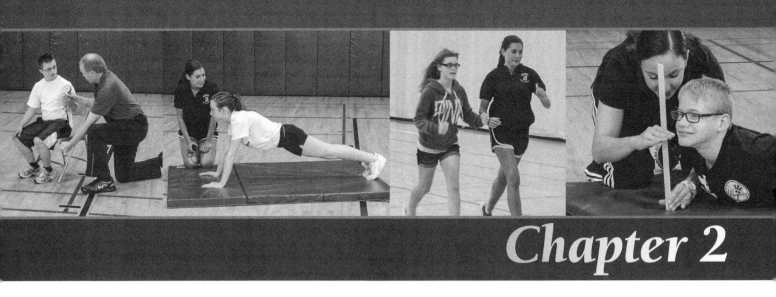

Chapter 2

The Conceptual Framework

The Brockport Physical Fitness Test (BPFT) is a criterion-referenced test of health-related fitness. In this criterion-referenced approach, test scores obtained by youngsters are compared with standards and fitness zones thought to be associated with an index of positive health. Test users should understand the bases for these standards when assessing a young person's performance.

The framework for developing the BPFT is represented visually in figure 2.1. This schematic, modified from a model described by Bouchard and Shephard (1994), is helpful in understanding how BPFT test items and standards were selected. The following sections of this chapter discuss relationships between the elements depicted in figure 2.1: physical activity, health, and health-related physical fitness.

Physical Activity

Physical activity consists of any bodily movement produced by skeletal muscle resulting in a substantial increase over resting energy expenditure (Bouchard & Shephard, 1994). Although physical activity includes work and domestic chores (Bouchard & Shephard, 1994), the Brockport approach focuses on the categories shown in figure 2.1: exercise, sport, training, dance, and play. These types of physical activity can be performed in different patterns as dictated by the var-

iables of frequency, intensity, and duration. In the Brockport approach, the primary role of physical activity is the conditioning benefit it provides in developing health-related physical fitness.

Health

Health has been defined as a "human condition with physical, social, and psychological dimensions, each characterized on a continuum with positive and negative poles. Positive health is associated with a capacity to enjoy life and to withstand challenges; it is not merely the absence of disease. Negative health is associated with morbidity and, in the extreme, with premature mortality" (Bouchard & Shephard, 1994, p. 84).

In the Brockport paradigm, health is conceived as consisting of two main parts: **physiological health** and **functional health**. Physiological health is related to an individual's organic well-being. Thus indexes of physiological health include traits or capacities associated with well-being, absence of disease or condition, or low risk of developing a disease or condition. Examples of indexes of good physiological health include appropriate body composition and aerobic capacity.

Functional health is related to an individual's physical capability. Thus indexes of functional health include the ability to perform important

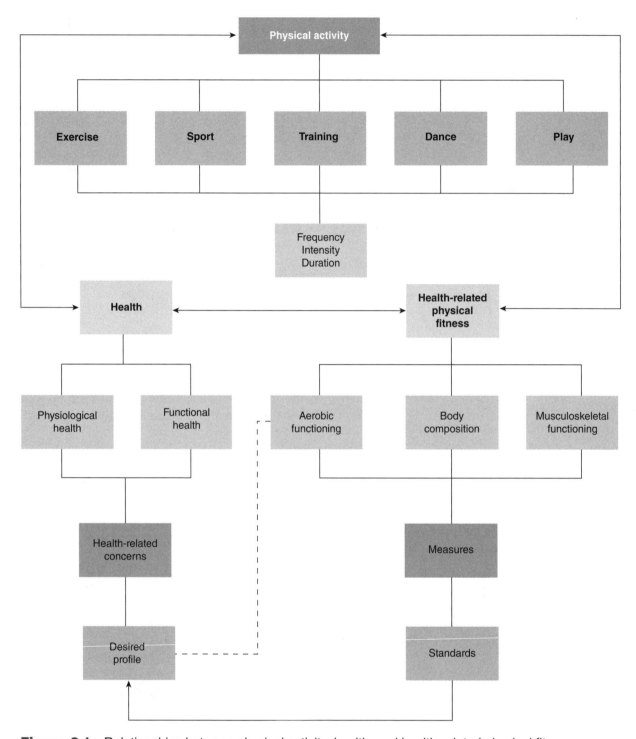

Figure 2.1 Relationships between physical activity, health, and health-related physical fitness.

Adapted, by permission, from C. Bouchard and R.J. Shephard, 1994, Physical activity, fitness, and health: The model and key concepts. In *Physical activity, fitness, and health: International proceedings and consensus statement*, edited by C. Bouchard, R.J. Shephard, and T. Stephens (Champaign, IL: Human Kinetics), 77-86.

tasks independently and to independently sustain such performance. Examples of indexes of good functional health include the ability to perform activities of daily living (ADLs), sustain physical activity, and participate in leisure activities.

Both physiological health and functional health contribute to a person's capacity to enjoy life and withstand challenges. Both also provide indexes of health that serve as bases for health-related physical fitness standards.

Health-Related Physical Fitness

The Brockport definition of **health-related physical fitness** is as follows:

> Health-related fitness refers to the components of fitness affected by habitual physical activity and related to health status. It is defined as a state characterized by (a) an ability to perform and sustain daily activities and (b) demonstration of traits or capacities associated with low risk of premature development of diseases and conditions related to movement (adapted from Pate, 1988).

The health-related components of fitness adopted for this test include aerobic functioning, body composition, and musculoskeletal functioning. **Aerobic functioning** encompasses both **aerobic capacity** (maximal oxygen uptake, or $\dot{V}O_2max$) and **aerobic behavior** (the ability to perform aerobic activity at specified levels of intensity and duration). **Body composition** provides an indication of the degree of body leanness or fatness (usually percent body fat). **Musculoskeletal functioning** combines muscular strength, muscular endurance, and flexibility or range of motion. The relationship of these elements is evident when combining them, especially when designing a fitness program. For example, improving the range of motion of a joint in a young person with a disability may require improving the extensibility of the agonistic muscle while improving the strength of the antagonistic muscle.

A Personalized Approach

Several identifiable characteristics are exhibited by field-based, norm-referenced, or criterion-referenced tests of physical fitness that have been developed and used with youngsters in the past few years. Important here is the fact that these tests have been developed largely on the basis of an assumed commonality of factors, such as physical fitness purposes, needs, test items, and standards. Individualization within tests has typically been limited to—and focused on—considerations related to age and gender. Thus tests have typically consisted of a selected number of items performed in a specific way and evaluated using a general population standard (e.g., a Healthy Fitness Zone). In addition, the tests have usually been developed *for* youngsters rather than *with* youngsters.

Although such tests clearly offer value for the hypothetical typical young person, they also clearly offer limited value for youngsters with disability. The health-related concerns of youngsters with disability may include, as well as differ from, those of youth in the general population. Specific disabilities may affect movement modes, movement abilities, and health-related physical fitness potential. For example, an individual who is completely paralyzed in the lower extremities and uses a wheelchair is unable to demonstrate aerobic functioning by running a mile. For such an individual, a different approach is needed for demonstrating and assessing aerobic functioning. Similarly, an individual with double-leg amputation at or near the hip joint requires different standards than peers without disability do for maximal oxygen intake and body mass index in order to validly evaluate fitness. Clearly, then, test items for measuring physical fitness may be different for youngsters with such disabilities. At times, health-related concerns and subcomponents of physical fitness also may need to be different from those selected for peers without disability.

Because of the wide variation in the needs and abilities of youngsters with disability, the specific nature of a physical fitness test should be developed, as much as possible, through personal association and interaction with the individuals being tested. Such interaction enables the test to be personalized as well as individualized—two qualities that have not traditionally played an important role in the development of physical fitness tests.

The BPFT, in contrast, has incorporated a personalized approach to physical fitness testing and assessment. After the development of a health-related, criterion-referenced physical fitness orientation and a corresponding definition of physical fitness, the following steps are suggested for personalizing a health-related, criterion-referenced physical fitness test:

- Identify and select health-related concerns of importance to the young person.

- Establish a desired, personalized fitness profile with (or, as necessary, for) the young person.
- Select components and subcomponents of physical fitness to be assessed.
- Select test items to measure the selected fitness components and subcomponents.
- Select criterion-referenced standards and fitness zones to evaluate the individual's physical fitness.

Each of these steps is discussed in the sections that follow.

Health-Related Concerns

After acceptance of a health-related physical fitness orientation, the first step in developing a personalized physical fitness test for a person or class of people is to identify and select health-related concerns that the test will address or emphasize. In practice, health concerns of the general population are reviewed to determine whether they are appropriate for youngsters with disability. These health concerns provide the basis for standards in which health status is the criterion. For example, the developers of Fitnessgram (Cooper Institute, 2010, 2013) have identified the following health-related concerns to be addressed by their test: high blood pressure, coronary heart disease, stroke, obesity, diabetes, some forms of cancer, lower-back flexibility, functional health, and other health problems.

These items may also be basic concerns of an individual with disability. However, individuals with disability may also have additional health-related concerns. For example, a young person with a spinal cord injury requiring a wheelchair for ambulation may have health-related concerns typical of youth without disability *and* other concerns such as the ability to sustain aerobic activity; range of motion or flexibility of the hips or upper body; and strength and endurance to lift and transfer the body independently, lift the body to prevent decubitus ulcers (pressure sores), or propel a wheelchair manually. Health-related concerns such as these may be drawn from professional literature, expert opinion, opinions of parents and youngsters themselves, and other

sources as deemed appropriate. The key is to identify and select health-related concerns most relevant and important to the individual. Possible health-related concerns for the target populations in the BPFT can be found in chapter 4.

Desired, Personalized Profile

Once health-related concerns are identified, a desired, personalized physical fitness profile is developed for a person or class of people. A desired profile establishes the direction or broad goals for a health-related physical fitness program. A profile statement can be written that implicitly or explicitly identifies the components of physical fitness to be addressed and expresses the underlying value of each component to the health-related concerns. The profile thus serves as a reference for a desired personal state of physical fitness. The profile also serves as a basis for the selection of test items and standards for evaluating health-related physical fitness. Desired profiles, in essence, are goals that require at least minimally acceptable levels of physical fitness. Examples of desired profiles for the target populations are provided in chapter 4.

Components of Physical Fitness

Components of physical fitness associated with the BPFT include aerobic functioning, body composition, and musculoskeletal functioning. Each of these components includes subcomponents that can be selected for a personalized physical fitness test. Within the component of aerobic functioning, for example, one can select the subcomponent aerobic capacity or that of aerobic behavior, or both, for a personalized physical fitness test. Subcomponents of body composition include percent body fat and the ratio of weight to height (body mass index). Subcomponents of musculoskeletal functioning include muscular strength, muscular endurance, and flexibility or range of motion. Components and subcomponents included in a personalized test should be consistent with the desired, personalized profile. The BPFT recommends that, to the extent possible, all three components of physical fitness be included in every personalized test of physical fitness.

Test Items

Once components and subcomponents of health-related physical fitness are selected in light of health-related concerns, test items are chosen to measure the selected components. The criteria to be used in selecting test items include validity, reliability, the extent of use for different classes of youngsters, the extent of information provided by a test item, economy of time and expense, user-friendliness, and feasibility in field situations.

Test Items by BPFT Fitness Component

- Aerobic functioning
  - PACER (20-meter and 15-meter)
  - One-mile run/walk
  - Target aerobic movement test (TAMT)
- Body composition
  - Percent body fat—skinfolds
  - Percent body fat—bioelectrical impedance analysis
  - Body mass index (BMI)
- Musculoskeletal functioning
  - Reverse curl
  - Seated push-up
  - 40-meter push/walk
  - Wheelchair ramp test
  - Push-up
  - Isometric push-up
  - Pull-up
  - Modified pull-up
  - Bench press
  - Dumbbell press
  - Dominant grip strength
  - Back-saver sit-and-reach
  - Flexed-arm hang
  - Extended-arm hang
  - Trunk lift
  - Curl-up
  - Modified curl-up
  - Target stretch test (TST)
  - Modified Apley test
  - Shoulder stretch
  - Modified Thomas test

Selection guides are provided in chapter 4 to help testers select the tests that are most appropriate for a young person with a particular disability. For more detailed information about validity and reliability, as well as background regarding the selection and attainability of standards, see the technical information presented by Winnick and Short (2005).

Standards and Fitness Zones for Evaluating Physical Fitness

Once test items have been selected to measure components and subcomponents of physical fitness, the next step is to develop Healthy Fitness Zones (HFZs) and adapted fitness zones (AFZs) based on both general and specific standards to serve as a basis for fitness evaluation from a health-status orientation.

Profiles, Test Items, Standards, and Fitness Zones

Personalization implies that once testers identify appropriate health-related concerns, they can write their own physical fitness profiles (in consultation with youngsters, where appropriate), select their own test items related to components of health-related fitness, and decide on their own standards. The BPFT provides information about profiles, items, and standards that testers can adopt, as appropriate, for use with youngsters.

The BPFT provides 10 profile statements related to three components of health-related fitness: aerobic functioning, body composition, and musculoskeletal functioning (see figures 2.2 through 2.6, located at the end of this chapter). Two profile statements each are given for aerobic functioning and body composition, and six are given for musculoskeletal functioning (four related primarily to strength and endurance and two to flexibility or range of motion). For each profile statement, test items and standards are recommended with the target populations in mind. Testers can select profiles, tests, and standards from the options provided. Testers always have the additional option to adjust or substitute material.

Figures 2.2 through 2.6 at the end of this chapter show relationships between fitness components, subcomponents, the 10 profile statements, test items, and standards. Standards are either general or specific. A **general standard** is a target measure of attainment associated with the general population. It is a test score related to acceptable functional or physiological health and is attainable by youngsters whose performance is not significantly limited by impairment. General standards are assumed to reflect minimal acceptable levels of health-related fitness and provide the basis for **Healthy Fitness Zones**. For most test items, the general standard is the lowest score one can make and still achieve the HFZ.

A **specific standard** may also reflect functional or physiological health, but it has been adjusted in some way to account for the performance effects of a specific impairment. Specific standards provide the basis for the Brockport Physical Fitness Test's **adapted fitness zones (AFZs)**. Ordinarily, the lowest boundary of an AFZ is defined by the specific standard, and the upper boundary of an AFZ is set by the general standard (i.e., the start of the HFZ). Specific standards reflect at least minimally acceptable levels of health-related fitness adjusted for the effects of disability. Specific standards can also reflect attainable levels of physical fitness leading to acceptable levels of health-related fitness.

An HFZ may be recommended for the general population and for certain youngsters with disability. AFZs are provided only for selected test items for specific target populations. For most recommended test items in the BPFT, a young person's test score generally falls into one of three assessment categories: needs improvement, adapted fitness zone, or Healthy Fitness Zone.

If a standard (or fitness zone) is not provided for a particular test item or is believed to be inappropriate for a specific young person, the tester is encouraged to develop **individualized standards** by which to assess performance. An individualized standard is a desired level of fitness for an individual that is established with consideration of the individual's present level of performance and expectation for progress. It is not necessarily a health-related standard. For a standard to be health-related, it must meet be linked (through research, logic, or expert opinion) to some index of positive health.

The BPFT presents three levels or fitness zones related to health-related fitness. The lowest level is designated as needs improvement. Individuals in this level need improvement in the specific area of fitness being measured. The second level, designated as an adapted fitness zone (AFZ), reflects a minimum acceptable level of health-related physical fitness adjusted for the effects of an impairment or an attainable level of physical fitness leading to a Healthy Fitness Zone. A specific standard is a target measure that serves as a basis for the AFZ. The third level, designated as a Healthy Fitness Zone (HFZ), reflects an acceptable level of health-related fitness that is associated with the general population not adjusted for impairment. The HFZ is based on a general standard.

The data for general and specific standards and associated fitness zones in the BPFT come from two sources: Fitnessgram (Cooper, 2013) for test items on the BPFT that are also on the Fitnessgram, and Project Target (Project Target, 1998) for BPFT test items not on Fitnessgram. The Fitnessgram test is a health-related physical fitness test designed primarily for youngsters without disabilities. Project Target was a federally funded project designed to provide data to develop specific and general standards for test items on the BPFT for youngsters with and without disabilities. This association of Fitnessgram and the BPFT enhances a close relationship between the tests. Such relationship is also addressed briefly in chapter 3.

The Basis for Standards

The BPFT includes 27 test items categorized under three components of health-related fitness. This large number of test items gives testers flexibility when personalizing the test. In most cases, testers select four to six test items to be used with a particular young person. The following sections discuss each of the test items, which are grouped by fitness component: aerobic functioning, body composition, and musculoskeletal functioning. For each item, the discussion also briefly addresses the bases for the associated criterion-referenced standards.

For an in-depth treatment of standards unique to the Brockport Physical Fitness Test, see Winnick and Short (2005). For more technical information, readers may also be interested in the *Fitnessgram/Activitygram Reference Guide* (Welk & Meredith, 2008), which relates to Fitnessgram test items and standards used in the Brockport test, and the *Fitnessgram and Activitygram Test Administration Manual* (Cooper Institute, 2010, 2013).

Aerobic Functioning

Aerobic functioning is the component of physical fitness that permits an individual to sustain large-muscle, dynamic, moderate- to high-intensity activity for prolonged periods of time. This component depends primarily on the efficiency or development of the heart, lung, blood, and skeletal muscle metabolic functions. Aerobic functioning is perhaps the most important of the health-related components of fitness because it relates clearly to both functional and physiological aspects of health. Adequate aerobic functioning allows a person to sustain physical activity for work, play, and emergencies; it may also reduce the risk of developing certain diseases.

In the BPFT, aerobic functioning has two separate but related subcomponents: aerobic capacity and aerobic behavior. A person's aerobic capacity is the highest rate at which he or she can consume oxygen while exercising—thus the more fit a person is, the greater his or her aerobic capacity. Good aerobic capacity enhances performance in endurance activities and is associated with reduced risk of developing certain diseases and conditions in adulthood, including high blood pressure, coronary heart disease, obesity, diabetes, and some forms of cancer. Aerobic capacity standards developed by Fitnessgram (Cooper Institute, 2013) and used in this test distinguish youngsters with and without metabolic syndrome risk factors associated with cardiovascular disease and diabetes.

The best measure of aerobic capacity is generally considered to be a laboratory measurement of maximal oxygen uptake ($\dot{V}O_2$max). General standards and HFZs for $\dot{V}O_2$max are based on Fitnessgram standards (Cooper Institute, 2013), which enable classification into three zones: Healthy

Fitness Zone (good health), needs improvement, and needs improvement (health risk).

Aerobic capacity can also be estimated in a field setting, and two such methods are used in the BPFT: the one-mile run/walk and the PACER (15-meter and 20-meter) performance test items. The mile run/walk formula includes body composition (BMI); the PACER formula does not. The equation used to predict $\dot{V}O_2$max from the mile run/walk derives from work by Cureton, Sloniger, O'Bannon, Black, and McCormack (1995). The equation is based on a sample of 753 males and females (aged 8 to 25 years) and uses age (in years), sex (coded as 0 for female or 1 for male), body mass index (BMI, in units of kilograms × meters[2]), and mile run/walk time (in minutes) for the prediction:

$$\dot{V}O_2\text{max} = (0.21 \times \text{age} \times \text{sex}) - (0.84 \times \text{BMI}) - (8.41 \times \text{time}) + (0.34 \times \text{time}^2) + 108.94$$

Thus, for a 14-year-old boy with a BMI of 22 and a mile run time of 9.07, the $\dot{V}O_2$max is 45.09 = (0.21 × 14) − (0.84 × 22) − (8.41 × 9.07) + (0.34 × 82.26) + 108.94.

Since this equation predicts $\dot{V}O_2$max using both mile run/walk time and BMI, it is not possible to represent the results solely by mile time in tabular form; therefore, the standards in chapter 4 are expressed not in minutes and seconds but in milliliters/kilograms/minutes. Furthermore, this equation cannot be used to calculate $\dot{V}O_2$max for mile run times above 13 minutes. Therefore, youngsters who cannot run a mile in 13 minutes or less need to take the PACER test to get an estimate of $\dot{V}O_2$max.

The equation for estimating $\dot{V}O_2$max from the 20-meter PACER comes from the Cooper Institute (2013): $\dot{V}O_2$max = 45.619 + (0.353 × 20-meter PACER laps) − (1.121 × age). (If the 15-meter PACER is used, the number of 15-meter laps is converted to an equivalent number of 20-meter laps for use in this $\dot{V}O_2$max formula. The lap conversion tables can be found in appendix D.) Thus, if a 12-year-old does 25 laps on the 20-meter PACER, his or her $\dot{V}O_2$max is 41.0 = 45.619 + (0.353 × 25) − (1.121 × 12).

It should be noted that BMI is not used to predict $\dot{V}O_2$max when using the PACER formula. For the BPFT, it is recommended that the PACER, rather than the mile run, be selected to calculate $\dot{V}O_2$max. First, since the mile run formula is not calculated or recommended if a youngster cannot complete the mile in 13 minutes, $\dot{V}O_2$max results *could be completed* using PACER data. Thus the PACER technique permits calculation for the shortest and slowest of performances, which is not the case using the mile run formula. This is a factor to consider since youngsters with disabilities often have shorter and slower performances. Second, since the PACER option does not require BMI in its calculation, users of the BPFT may consult tables in chapter 4 to offer lap targets to attain specific levels of fitness even prior to testing. Finally, the PACER option reduces poor performers from the embarrassment associated with finishing last in a mile run setting.

Aerobic capacity standards in the BPFT are sometimes adjusted to reflect disability-specific concerns. For instance, youngsters who are blind may need to participate in running items with some form of tactual assistance or guidance (e.g., guide wire, sighted partner). Running with such an encumbrance requires more energy than running unassisted. Consequently, specific aerobic capacity standards for runners who require tactual assistance are 3 percent lower than general standards in order to account for the higher energy demands of their activity. For those who run with assistance, the specific criterion-referenced standards are meant to be consistent with the recommendation made by Buell (1983), which called for a reduction in performance standards on distance runs for youngsters who are blind and require assistance. In addition, because running inefficiency is believed to influence performance, assisted blind runners who attain general standards likely possess levels of aerobic capacity greater than those of students in the general population.

Youngsters with intellectual disability may also require adjustment of $\dot{V}O_2$max standards. As a result, in the original version of the BPFT, with the help of a panel of experts, the specific PACER lap standards were based on a 10 percent downward adjustment in accompanying $\dot{V}O_2$max values (Winnick & Short, 2005). That is, specific PACER lap standards were predicted from $\dot{V}O_2$max scores that were 10 percent below those recommended for the general population. This approach was not intended to suggest that it is acceptable for youngsters with intellectual disability to have $\dot{V}O_2$max values below those of the general population; it is not. Rather, the 10 percent downward adjustment was meant to account for the movement inefficiencies (due to maturational delay, incoordination, smaller body size, or other factors) that likely suppress PACER test performance in many youngsters with intellectual disability. These suppressed test scores, in turn, would result in underestimated $\dot{V}O_2$max values.

This premise is carried forward in this edition of the BPFT. The general standards for aerobic capacity are the Healthy Fitness Zone standards adopted from the 2013 version of Fitnessgram, and the specific standards and corresponding AFZs for youngsters with intellectual disability are derived by reducing those general standards by 10 percent. Test users are cautioned, however, that the specific standards for individuals with intellectual disability are not necessarily associated with indexes of health-related fitness (i.e., a young person with intellectual disability may achieve the AFZ but still be at risk for certain fitness-related diseases and conditions). Whenever possible, youngsters with intellectual disability should be encouraged to pursue the general standards and HFZs, but for many youngsters with intellectual disability, the AFZs provide a more realistic, but still challenging, intermediate target.

In some cases, it is not yet possible to estimate aerobic capacity accurately in a field setting. Making such an estimate is particularly problematic for those with physical disability, especially cerebral palsy. The complexity of making an estimate depends on the extent and nature of impairment, the type of any wheelchair or other assistive device used, and the type of surface on which the test is conducted. There is also some belief, which we share, that functional health-related needs represented by aerobic behavior are relevant and important to the individual and can be more accurately and feasibly measured than aerobic capacity in field-based tests for people with disability. For these reasons, a measure of aerobic *capacity* is not recommended for certain youngsters with disability; what is suggested instead is a measure of aerobic *behavior*.

The term aerobic behavior refers to the ability to sustain physical activity of a specific intensity for a particular duration. The measure of aerobic behavior associated with the BPFT is the target aerobic movement test (TAMT). Individuals who demonstrate the ability to sustain moderate physical activity for 15 minutes meet the general standard for health-related aerobic behavior. Moderate exercise involves a heart rate of at least 70 percent of maximal predicted heart rate, adjusted for disability or mode of exercise. The TAMT has two criteria—one for intensity and one for duration. The ability to sustain at least moderate-level activity for 15 minutes has positive implications for functional health, especially for ADLs and participation in leisure-time pursuits (including games and sports). Furthermore, when performed regularly, this level of activity is believed to be consistent with existing general recommendations for enhancing or maintaining health.

See chapter 4 for a description of adjustments made to general standards for BPFT test items associated with both aerobic capacity and aerobic behavior for populations with specific disabilities.

Body Composition

Body composition is the component of health-related physical fitness that involves the body's degree of leanness or fatness. It has implications for both functional health and physiological health. When fat levels in the body are too high, a person's ability to lift or move the body is negatively affected. Similarly, obesity has been found to be associated with an increased risk of diabetes, coronary heart disease, high blood pressure, arthritis, various forms of cancer, and all-cause mortality (U.S. Department of Health and Human Services, 1996).

The measures of body composition used in the BPFT include skinfolds, bioelectrical impedance analysis, and body mass index. Percent body fat indicates the proportion of body weight that is fat, whereas **body mass index (BMI)** estimates the appropriateness of weight for height. Skinfold sites used to predict percent body fat in the BPFT include triceps plus calf (TC), triceps plus subscapular (TS), and triceps only (TO). The selection of sites for skinfold measurement can be affected by individual factors (e.g., body braces or missing limbs).

BMI scores for youngsters with disability must be interpreted carefully. Results may be invalidated by underestimates of either height (e.g., due to contractures at the knees or hips) or weight (e.g., due to a missing limb or loss of active muscle mass).

Body composition is assessed by using 2013 Fitnessgram standards. Percent body fat in young people is classified into zones associated with degree of health risk and level of fitness: healthy fitness (good health), needs improvement, and needs improvement (health risk). A fourth zone—very lean—suggests that there are also health-related concerns associated with excessive leanness or thinness. BMI standards are equated with corresponding values for percent body fat, and standards for both BMI and percent body fat vary by age and gender. No disability-specific standards for body composition are selected for individuals in the BPFT; general standards associated with HFZs are recommended for all youngsters.

Musculoskeletal Functioning

Musculoskeletal functioning combines three traditional components of physical fitness: **muscular strength**, **muscular endurance**, and **flexibility** or **range of motion**. The relationship between musculoskeletal functioning and health (especially functional health) has a logical basis. Certain levels of strength, endurance, and flexibility are necessary to maintain good posture, live independently, and participate in leisure-time activities.

Measures of musculoskeletal functioning, primarily muscular strength and muscular endurance, include the bench press, dumbbell press, extended-arm hang, flexed-arm hang, dominant grip strength, push-up, isometric push-up, pull-up, modified pull-up, curl-up, modified curl-up, and trunk lift. Although each of these test items can be justified on the basis of logical validity, no specific level of strength or endurance has been identified as critical for health. Instead, criterion-referenced standards associated with these items are based primarily on expert opinion (Plowman & Corbin, 1994; Plowman, 2008). The goal for the general standard associated with some of these tests is to score at or above the 20th percentile for the general population.

Specific standards and AFZs for some muscular strength and muscular endurance items are provided for youngsters with intellectual disability and mild limitations in fitness. The literature consistently documents a performance discrepancy between youngsters with intellectual disability and those without on many measures of muscular strength and muscular endurance. In attempting to explain the performance gap, researchers have cited factors such as motivation, fewer opportunities to train, fewer opportunities to participate in physical activity, poor instruction, and physiological factors. With this gap in mind, where specific standards and an AFZ are provided in the BPFT for youngsters with intellectual disability, they are lower than the general and HFZ standards by a range of 25 percent to 50 percent. The percentage used for a specific item is an estimate of the performance discrepancy identified for that item in previous research. Specific standards associated with AFZs are 50 percent of general standards for the isometric push-up, flexed-arm hang, and bench press; 60 percent for the curl-ups; 65 percent for grip strength; and 75 percent for the extended-arm hang.

For youngsters with *physical* disability, no specific standards are provided for these measures of muscular strength and endurance. It is, however, especially important to select appropriate test items for these individuals. Youngsters with some form of paraplegia (due to either cerebral palsy or spinal cord injury) should be able to achieve general standards for upper-body measures involving the hands or arms but may have difficulty with measures involving the trunk or abdomen. Unilateral test items (e.g., dominant grip strength and dumbbell press) have the most relevance for youngsters with some types of cerebral palsy, particularly hemiplegia, and for those with single-limb amputation.

Muscular strength and muscular endurance can also be assessed by means of the reverse curl, seated push-up, and 40-meter push/walk, which are most appropriate for youngsters with certain types of physical disability. Bases for specific standards for these items derive from their relationship to ADLs. The specific standard for the reverse curl, for instance, is tied directly to the functional ability to lift a 1-pound (0.5-kilogram) weight one time. It is assumed that such an ability carries functional significance for youngsters who are more severely disabled (especially those with low-level cervical spinal cord injury) and who might hope to lift a lightweight object in performing ADLs.

The specific standards for the seated push-up are selected on the basis of two possibilities. The 5-second standard relates to the recommendation that wheelchair users relieve the skin pressure on their buttocks and legs for about 5 seconds every 15 minutes. Such a regimen is believed to reduce the risk of developing decubitus ulcers (Kosiak & Kottke, 1990). The 20-second specific standard for the seated push-up would be selected if health concerns related to other ADLs (e.g., transferring) require longer strength or endurance performance.

The basis for the specific standard for the 40-meter push/walk is the potential for functional mobility. The minimal value for functional walking speed in adults is approximately 40 meters per minute (Waters, 1992). This value has been adopted as the specific standard, provided that it can be attained at a heart rate of 125 beats per minute or less (see adjustments for disability in the description of this test item in chapter 5). If a young person can travel at 40 meters per minute at this light intensity, it is assumed that he or she can maintain that functional speed over longer distances required for the performance of ADLs in the community.

The standards for the wheelchair ramp test are related to the American National Standards Institute (ANSI) recommendation that ramps be constructed with an incline ratio of 12 inches (30 centimeters) of run for every inch (2.5 centimeters) of rise in elevation. Thus a ramp built to negotiate a 2-foot (0.6-meter) elevation must be 24 feet (7.3 meters) long. For the ramp test, two possibilities exist for specific standards. The first—a standard of 8 feet (2.4 meters) of run—is linked to the ability to ascend 8 inches (20 centimeters) of elevation, or the height of approximately one step. Stair steps have a uniform height of 7 inches (18 centimeters), and curb cuts have a maximum rise of 8 inches. The second specific standard— referred to as the 15-foot (4.6-meter) standard—is actually a floating standard that can be matched to the length of a ramp (up to 30 feet, or 9.1 meters) that the young person may encounter on a daily basis. That is, testers may set this standard anywhere between 15 and 30 feet, depending on the mobility demands faced by the young person on a daily basis.

Tests of flexibility or range of motion include the shoulder stretch, modified Apley test, modified Thomas test, back-saver sit-and-reach, and target stretch test (TST). The shoulder stretch and modified Apley test both measure shoulder flexibility. The shoulder stretch test is justified solely on a logical basis. It provides only two result options: pass or fail. A passing score is given when a youngster meets the general standard and displays HFZ-optimal shoulder flexibility.

In contrast, the modified Apley test is scored on a scale of 0 to 3, wherein 3 indicates optimal shoulder flexibility; 2 suggests enough shoulder flexibility to potentially perform functional activities such as washing, combing the hair, or removing a cap; 1 indicates the potential to perform functional activities such as eating and brushing the teeth; and 0 means insufficient flexibility to accomplish any of the listed tasks. A score of 3 is the general standard, and it is expected that most youngsters can achieve it. Specific standards are provided only for youngsters with more severe forms of cerebral palsy (classes C1 and C2).

The modified Thomas test measures hip flexibility but is recommended only for ambulatory individuals. Scores are tied to the extent of limitation in the hip flexors: a score of 3 indicates optimal hip extension, 2 suggests some tightness in the hip flexors that results in an approximately 15-degree or smaller loss in range of motion, 1 indicates a loss of about 15 to 30 degrees, and 0 indicates a loss of more than about 30 degrees. The general standard is 3. A specific standard is provided only for youngsters with a type of cerebral palsy that typically restricts hip flexibility (class C5 and C7 for the affected side).

The back-saver sit-and-reach test has been shown to validly measure hamstring flexibility. Sit-and-reach tests have been included in health-related fitness test batteries for a number of years because of a presumed relationship to low-back pain. Although research evidence has yet to confirm this relationship, anatomical logic

for it is strong. Only HFZ levels based on general standards are provided in this manual. As with many test items for muscular strength and muscular endurance, the standards for the back-saver sit-and-reach test are based on expert opinion (Plowman & Corbin, 1994).

The target stretch test (TST) is a subjective measure of movement extent that can be applied to a number of joint actions. Individualized standards (those developed by testers for young people's specific needs) are recommended for some youngsters. For most, however, the basis for the specific standard is to have functional range of motion on at least one side of the body. Functional range of motion is represented by a score of 1 on the test; the Project Target Advisory Committee considered this a clinically acceptable level of range of motion that is typically obtainable and meets minimal AFZ requirements for functional activity. The general standard, represented by a score of 2, depicts optimal range of motion for a particular joint. Individuals who are free of physical impairment should strive for an optimal HFZ level on the TST.

Sources of Standards and Fitness Zones

Standards recommended in the BPFT are derived from a variety of sources. Several criterion-referenced, health-related standards and Healthy Fitness Zones appropriate for the general population—and sometimes recommended for youngsters with disability—were developed for Fitnessgram by the Cooper Institute for Aerobics Research (1992, 1999) and the Cooper Institute (2010, 2013). The 2013 standards and Healthy Fitness Zones are used in this edition of the BPFT. These are the same standards employed in the Fitnessgram program, and their application is presented in chapter 4. They include standards for the following items: $\dot{V}O_2$max, percent body fat, body mass index, curl-up, trunk lift, push-up, pull-up, modified pull-up, flexed-arm hang, back-saver sit-and-reach, and shoulder stretch.

Standards reflecting HFZ performance of the general population for items not associated with Fitnessgram were developed on the basis of data collected on 913 youngsters from the Brockport

(New York) Central School District as part of Project Target. Standards related to performance of the general population on the dumbbell press, bench press, extended-arm hang, dominant grip strength, and isometric push-up were based in part on these data and are acknowledged as Project Target data in chapter 4. General standards and HFZ levels for the modified Apley, modified Thomas, target stretch, and target aerobic movement tests were based on expert opinion (Project Target Advisory Committee, 1997).

Specific standards were also based on expert opinion, related literature, and data from samples of youngsters with disability. Data collected as part of Project Target were used to field-test the suitability, attainability, and reliability of—and the standards for—the following tests: bench press, extended-arm hang, flexed-arm hang, modified curl-up, dominant grip strength, isometric push-up, seated push-up, reverse curl, 40-meter push/walk, modified Apley and Thomas tests, PACER, and one-mile run/walk. Data associated with Project UNIQUE (Winnick & Short, 1985) were also consulted in selecting standards for the flexed-arm hang, dominant grip strength, and skinfold measures. Recommended specific standards for youngsters with intellectual disability were developed by consulting data provided by Eichstaedt, Polacek, Wang, and Dohrman (1991); Hayden (1964); and the Canada Fitness Award (Government of Canada, Fitness and Amateur Sport, 1985). Standards associated with the TST are based on optimal levels of range of motion presented by Cole and Tobis (1990), and functional standards were recommended by the Project Target Advisory Committee (1997).

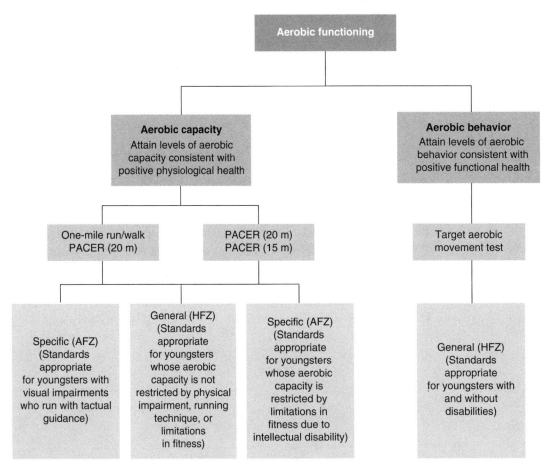

Figure 2.2 Profiles, test items, standards, and zones related to aerobic functioning.

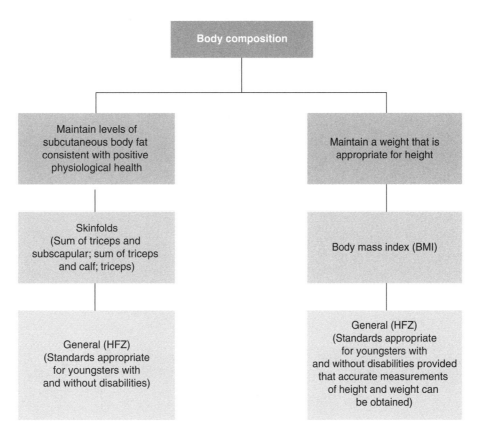

Figure 2.3 Profiles, test items, standards, and zones related to body composition.

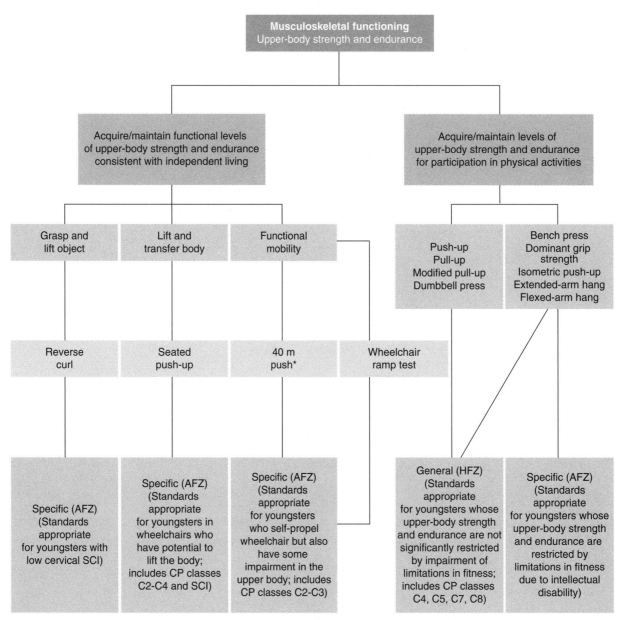

* 40 m push is used as a general strength and endurance item.

Figure 2.4 Profiles, test items, standards, and zones related to upper-body strength and endurance.

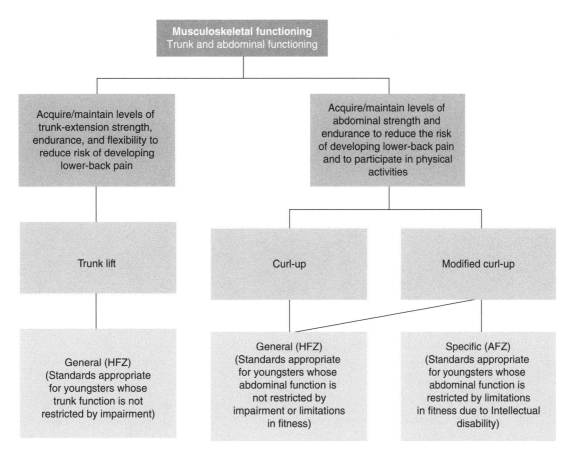

Figure 2.5 Profiles, test items, standards, and zones related to trunk and abdominal functioning.

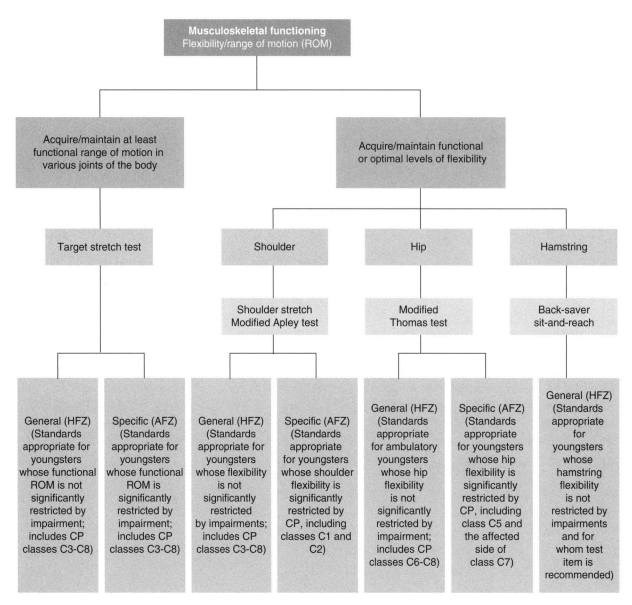

Figure 2.6 Profiles, test items, standards, and zones related to flexibility or range of motion.

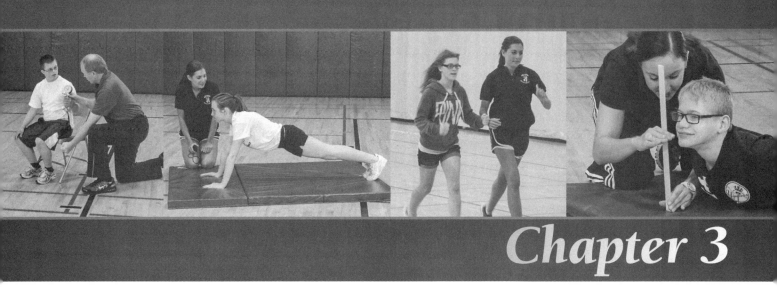

Chapter 3

Using the Brockport Physical Fitness Test

This test manual presents both the Brockport Physical Fitness Test (BPFT) and a process for modifying the test for young people with unique needs. It suggests profile statements, components of fitness, test items, standards, and fitness zones for youngsters in targeted populations. These fitness parameters are recommended based on information found in the professional literature or expressed by experts in the field. However, the health-related needs of a particular individual may vary from those of others in a particular group and may require adjustments in the parameters.

This chapter provides general information about how to test and evaluate using the BPFT, and it distinguishes three uses of the BPFT: (1) general procedures, (2) adjustments to general procedures for youngsters with disability, and (3) use of the BPFT with other tests. The final section of the chapter briefly addresses the development of an individualized education program (IEP).

General Procedures for Testing and Evaluating Physical Fitness

The most common way of using the BPFT is for testers to adopt the parameters recommended for use with youngsters who have specific disabilities. Though such an approach may not follow the practice of personalization in the strictest sense, it offers a number of advantages. First, because the parameters were developed with specific target populations in mind, they are likely to be relevant for a young person in a particular group. Second, each test item included in the battery is considered a valid and reliable health-related measure for members of the target population. Third, standards and fitness zones are recommended partly on the basis of field testing of subjects from the various target populations. Finally, adopting recommended parameters saves the tester time in personalizing the test.

Testers who choose to use the BPFT in this fashion follow a four-step process when administering the test:

1. Accurately classify or subclassify each young person.
2. Select appropriate test items.
3. Administer the chosen test items to measure physical fitness status.
4. Evaluate health-related physical fitness against recommended standards.

The tester's first responsibility is to accurately classify the young person to be tested according to the relevant disability (e.g., spinal cord injury, blindness). For youngsters with physical disability, the tester must also subclassify them according to the nature and extent of their disability. In order to complete this task, testers will probably need to consult the Target Populations section in chapter 1.

Once the young person is classified (and, as necessary, subclassified), the tester undertakes the second major step of the process—using the test-item selection guides (see the relevant tables in chapter 4) to choose test items. When selecting test items in this manner, the tester is implicitly adopting the desired profile written for a specific disability group, because the items were derived from the profile statements.

Some test items are recommended, whereas others are optional. A **recommended test item** relates to a particular component of physical fitness and a specific profile statement and is generally believed to be the best test of those parameters for a particular class of youngsters. Thus a recommended item is considered the first choice—but not necessarily the only choice—in test selection. Optional items also address specific components and profile statements, and they provide additional choices for testers. A tester might select an optional item over a recommended item for any number of reasons, such as equipment availability, facility requirements, the young person's individual characteristics, and the specific purpose for testing.

Regardless of whether a tester chooses recommended or optional items, the test battery ordinarily consists of four to six test items: one for aerobic functioning, one for body composition, and two to four for musculoskeletal functioning. Table 3.1 summarizes recommended and **optional test items**, as well as available standards, for each target population.

The tester's third responsibility is to measure the individual's physical fitness status by administering the chosen test items appropriately. This process is addressed in detail in chapter 5, which provides recommendations for test administration, including necessary equipment, scoring, trials, test modifications, and safety guidelines and precautions. After administering the chosen test items, the tester records the results; experi-enced testers may develop recording systems that work best for them.

The tester's final responsibility is to evaluate the health-related physical fitness level of each young person. Individuals are evaluated by comparing their results on recommended or optional test items with criterion-referenced standards and fitness zones appropriate for them. The standards themselves appear in Fitness Zone tables 3 through 12 in chapter 4.

Both general and specific standards may be available to testers evaluating the physical fitness of youngsters with specific disabilities. General standards are available for almost all test items and are recommended when expectations for performance are typical of those for the general population—that is, when it is believed that a disability does not result in a unique physical fitness need and does not significantly alter performance expectations for the young person. Specific standards are available only for selected items where it is believed that a particular disability dictates an adjustment of general standards for a particular test (or when the test item is unique to a particular disability).

Testers should not assume that general standards are unattainable by a young person in a specific disability category. In fact, testers are encouraged to pursue general standards, even if specific standards are available, when the general standards are believed to be most appropriate or attainable by a particular young person.

Evaluating health-related fitness involves interpreting results and identifying unique needs, if any. Identified needs may be incorporated into a young person's individualized education program (IEP). For example, figure 3.1 presents a physical fitness profile sheet that might be developed for a young person, and figure 3.2 presents a sample summary of physical fitness data and a profile for a 14-year-old with an intellectual disability. Testers should compare past and current test results to track changes over time. Chapter 2 should be consulted for an explanation of standards and fitness zones.

Adjusting the BPFT

Although the recommended fitness parameters are likely to pertain to most youngsters in a specific

Table 3.1 Summary of Recommended and Optional Test Items With Available Standards

	General population		Intellectual disability		Blind with assistance		Cerebral palsy		Spinal cord injury		Congenital anomaly or amputation	
	Test item	Available standard	Test item	Available standard	Test item	Available standard	Test item	Available standard	Test item	Available standard	Test item	Available standard
AEROBIC FUNCTIONING												
PACER (20 m)	O	G	R†	S	R	S					R	G
PACER (15 m)	O	G	R†	S	R	S					R†	G
1-mile run/walk	R	G			O†	S					O†	G
TAMT	O	G*	R†	G*	O	G*	R	G*	R	G*	R†	G*
BODY COMPOSITION												
Percent fat	R	G	R	G	R	G	R	G	R	G	R	G
Skinfolds	R	G	R	G	R	G	R	G	R	G	R	G
BMI	O	G	O	G	O	G	O	G				
MUSCULOSKELETAL FUNCTIONING												
Reverse curl									R†	S*		
Seated push-up							R†	S	R†	S*	R†	S*
40 m push/walk							R†	S*				
Wheelchair ramp test							R†/O†	S*			R†	G
Bench press		G	O	S					O†	G		
Dumbbell press		G					R†/O†	G	O†	G	R†/O†	G
Extended-arm hang		G	R†	S								
Flexed-arm hang	O	G	R†	S	O	G						
Dominant grip strength		G	O	S			O†	G	R†	G	O†	G
Isometric push-up		G	O†	S								
Push-up	R	G			R	G						
Pull-up	O	G			O	G						
Modified pull-up	O	G			O	G						
Curl-up	R	G	R	S	R	G					R†	G
Modified curl-up												
Trunk lift	R	G*	R	G*	R	G*	R†	G/S*			R†	G*
Modified Apley test	O	G*					R†	G/S*	R†	G*	R†	G*
Shoulder stretch	O	G*	O	G*	O	G*			R†	G*	R†	G*
Modified Thomas test		G*					R†	G/S*	R†	G*		
Back-saver sit-and-reach	R	G*	R	G*	R	G*	R†/O†	G/S*			R†	G*
TST		G							R†	G*	R†	G*

Abbreviations: R = recommended item, O = optional item, G = general standard, and S = specific standard.

Note: "Blind with assistance" refers to youngsters who are blind and are being assisted in running activities.

*Only single (general or specific) standard is available.

†Item is recommended, or optional, for some (but not all) members of the category. (Consult test item selection guides in chapter 4.)

Physical Fitness Profile Sheet 👆

Name: _____ Date: _____

Gender: ____ M ____ F Age: _____ Disability: _____

Disability classification: _____

Physical fitness profile: Considering the health-related needs of this young person, construct a profile by placing check marks beside the statements that are most relevant to the individual's fitness needs. Then select specific test items and standards for measurement and assessment.

Aerobic Functioning

Aerobic Capacity

_____ Attain levels of aerobic capacity consistent with positive physiological health.

Aerobic Behavior

_____ Attain levels of aerobic behavior consistent with positive functional health.

Body Composition

Percent Body Fat

_____ Maintain levels of percent body fat consistent with positive physiological health.

Body Mass Index

_____ Maintain a weight that is appropriate for height.

Musculoskeletal Functioning

Strength and Endurance

_____ Acquire or maintain functional levels of upper-body strength and endurance consistent with independent living: (a) ability to grasp and lift a light weight, (b) ability to lift and transfer the body from a wheelchair, and/or (c) ability to attain functional mobility.

_____ Acquire or maintain levels of upper-body strength and endurance for participation in physical activities.

_____ Acquire or maintain levels of trunk-extension strength, endurance, and flexibility to reduce the risk of developing lower-back pain.

_____ Acquire or maintain levels of abdominal strength and endurance to reduce the risk of developing lower-back pain and to participate in physical activities.

Flexibility or Range of Motion

_____ Acquire or maintain at least functional range of motion in various joints.

_____ Acquire or maintain functional levels or optimal levels of flexibility in one or more of the following body regions: shoulders, hips, hamstrings.

From J. Winnick and F. Short, 2014, *Brockport physical fitness test manual: A health-related assessment for youngsters with disabilities* (Champaign, IL: Human Kinetics).

Figure 3.1 Sample physical fitness profile sheet.

Sample Physical Fitness Data Summary and Profile

Name: _____Jim Mayberry_____ Gender: _X_ M __ F Age: __14__

Height: _69 in. [1.75 m]_ Weight: _150 lb. [68 kg]_ Date: _Feb. 17, 2014_

Classification: _intellectual disability_ Subclassification: _n/a_

Aerobic Functioning

Test item	Unit of measure	Score	Adapted Fitness Zone (if applicable)	Healthy Fitness Zone
AEROBIC BEHAVIOR				
TAMT	min.	Pass	None	Pass

Body Composition

Test item	Unit of measure	Score	Adapted Fitness Zone (if applicable)	Healthy Fitness Zone
Sum of triceps and calf skinfolds	mm	27	None	8–28
Body mass index	BMI	22	None	16.4–23.0

Musculoskeletal Functioning

Test item	Unit of measure	Score	Adapted Fitness Zone (if applicable)	Healthy Fitness Zone
STRENGTH AND ENDURANCE				
Dominant grip	kg	25	22–32	≥33
Flexed-arm hang	sec.	6	08–14	≥15
Modified curl-up	#	16	14–23	≥24
FLEXIBILITY OR RANGE OF MOTION				
Back-saver sit-and-reach (right)	in.	8	None	8
Back-saver sit-and-reach (left)	in.	8	None	8
Trunk lift	in.	9	None	9–12

Interpretation: Meets Healthy Fitness Zones (HFZs) for aerobic behavior, flexibility, and body composition; below HFZ for dominant grip and modified curl-up; meets adapted fitness zones (AFZs) for dominant grip and modified curl-up; below AFZ standard for flexed-arm hang.

Needs: Priorities—Development of upper-body strength/endurance and abdominal strength/endurance.

Figure 3.2 Sample physical fitness data summary and profile.

target population, they may not be appropriate for all. Thus, when using the BPFT, testers always have latitude to adjust the parameters to meet a young person's unique needs. Testers may choose to delete, alter, or substitute for profile statements related to components of fitness, test items, or standards.

For instance, a tester might wish to use the model presented in figure 3.1 as a way of personalizing desired profiles for individual young people. Consider a teacher working with a boy who has a mild form of cerebral palsy. The teacher reviews the fitness parameters recommended for youngsters with cerebral palsy (see chapter 4) and decides to adopt the recommended profile, items, and standards. However, the teacher would also like to include a measure of abdominal strength and endurance for this young person, even though such a statement is not included in the recommended profile. The teacher could design a new profile by checking all the relevant profile statements in figure 3.1, including "Acquire or maintain levels of abdominal strength and endurance to reduce the risk of developing lower-back pain and to participate in physical activities." The teacher then selects test items measuring trunk and abdominal functioning (curl-ups or modified curl-ups, in this case) and either adopts the recommended standards available for the test or creates individualized standards for this young person.

In some cases, even if the recommended profile is appropriate for a particular young person, the recommended or optional test items might not be the best option. Consider, for example, a girl who is blind and also has an impairment that results in significant loss of function in her right arm. For youngsters who are blind, the push-up test of upper-body strength and endurance is recommended, but the teacher in this case believes it is inappropriate for this student. Instead, the teacher selects an alternative measure of upper-body strength and endurance that can be performed using just one side of the body (i.e., dumbbell press or dominant grip strength). The teacher properly decides to use the general standards to assess the strength and endurance of this young person's left hand or arm.

Whenever testers adjust the general procedures, they are encouraged to use the schematics presented in figures 2.2 through 2.6 in chapter 2 as a basis for changing profiles, items, or standards. Of course, testers are also free to develop their own fitness parameters as they deem necessary, but when they do so they should carefully document the parameters, including the bases for the standards.

Using the BPFT With Other Tests

Youngsters with disability are often able to perform one or more of the same test items and achieve the same performance standards as youngsters in the general population. Therefore, teachers in inclusive settings, for example, are encouraged to administer the test items from their regular test battery to students both with and without disability, when appropriate. There may be times, however, when either the test or the standards need to be different for a young person with a disability. In these circumstances, the BPFT can serve as a reference for filling in gaps in a testing program for a particular young person. Teachers who use Fitnessgram as their regular test battery will find it relatively easy to substitute items, standards, or both from the BPFT because of similarities between these two tests. And regardless of the test that a teacher uses, the BPFT can be used as a resource for personalization.

Developing an Individualized Education Program

Teachers should recognize that the BPFT's personalized approach is consistent with requirements for developing an individualized education program (IEP). Specifically, profile statements, with any necessary modifications, can be viewed as annual goals for a student's physical fitness. Recent test scores obtained by a young person can serve as entries in the present level of performance section of the IEP. General or specific standards and fitness zones can be consulted by the teacher and adopted or modified as performance criteria associated with short-term instructional objectives.

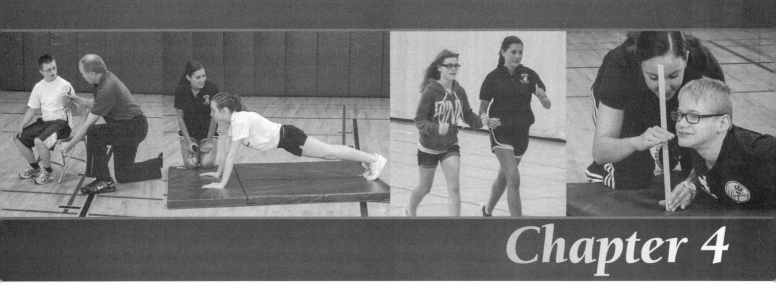

Profiles, Test Selection Guides, Standards, and Fitness Zones

This chapter presents the following elements: health-related, criterion-referenced parameters; test selection guides; standards; and fitness zones for assessing physical fitness for the general population and for each of the populations with disability targeted by the Brockport Physical Fitness Test. The chapter includes a series of tables depicting standards and fitness zones.

Index of Profiles

Cerebral palsy, page 37

Congenital anomaly or amputation, page 39

General population, page 30

Intellectual disability and mild limitations in physical fitness, page 31

Spinal cord injury, page 35

Visual impairment, page 33

Youngsters in the General Population

Health-Related Concerns

Health-related needs and concerns of youngsters in the general population include avoiding high blood pressure, coronary heart disease, obesity, diabetes, and some forms of cancer; maintaining lower-back health; and maintaining functional health.

Desired Profile

Boys and girls aged 10 to 17 years should possess, at minimum, levels of maximal oxygen uptake and body composition consistent with positive health, flexibility for functional health (especially good functioning of the lower back and hamstrings), and levels of abdominal and upper-body strength and endurance adequate for independent living and participation in physical activities.

Components of Physical Fitness

The components of physical fitness are categorized as aerobic functioning, body composition, and musculoskeletal functioning. Test items to assess these components appear in table 4.1.

Table 4.1 Test-Item Selection Guide for Youngsters in the General Population

Fitness component	Test item	Selection guide
Aerobic functioning	SELECT ONE:	
	1-mile run/walk (aerobic capacity)	R
	20 m PACER (aerobic capacity; strongly recommended for elementary and recommended for all ages)	R
	15 m PACER (aerobic capacity; strongly recommended for elementary)	R
	TAMT (aerobic behavior, level 1)	O
Body composition	SELECT ONE:	
	Percent body fat	R
	Skinfolds—sum of triceps and calf	R
	Body mass index	O
Musculoskeletal functioning	SELECT TWO:	
	Curl-up	R
	Trunk lift	R
	SELECT ONE:	
	90° push-up	R
	Modified pull-up	O
	Pull-up	O
	Flexed-arm hang	O
	SELECT ONE:	
	Back-saver sit-and-reach	R
	Shoulder stretch	O

Abbreviations: R = recommended; O = optional.
Data from The Cooper Institute 2013.

Standards and Fitness Zones

Standards and Healthy Fitness Zones (HFZs) from Fitnessgram for the general population are presented in Fitness Zone tables 1 and 2.

Aerobic Functioning

For the general population, aerobic capacity (via the PACER or one-mile run/walk) is evaluated using the HFZs from Fitnessgram. The aerobic capacity standards establish three zones based on potential risk for future health problems. Aerobic behavior, on the other hand, is measured using the target aerobic movement test (TAMT). It is evaluated using the HFZ based on general standards developed as part of Project Target (1998).

Body Composition

For the general population, body composition is evaluated using the standards and HFZs from Fitnessgram. Percent body fat is estimated using skinfolds (or bioelectrical impedance analysis). Body mass index (BMI) data corresponding to percentage fat for boys and girls in each targeted age group also come from Fitnessgram. "Boys and girls have BMI values that are very different due to the dramatic changes in growth and development that occur with age. Therefore, age- and sex-specific values of BMI are used to assess weight status for youth" (Cooper Institute, 2013, p. 43). The body composition standards establish four zones based on potential risks for future health problems.

Musculoskeletal Functioning

General standards from Fitnessgram for muscular strength and endurance items are used to evaluate youngsters in the general population. Minimal muscular strength and endurance standards correspond closely to fitness levels equal to those for the 20th percentile of the general population. General standards from Fitnessgram associated with test items designed to assess flexibility (back-saver sit-and-reach and shoulder stretch) or trunk extension strength and flexibility (trunk lift) are based on normative data and expert judgment on what represents an acceptable level of function. For the trunk lift, scores beyond 12 inches (30 centimeters) are discouraged.

Youngsters With Intellectual Disability and Mild Limitations in Physical Fitness

Health-Related Concerns

Health-related needs and concerns of youngsters with intellectual disability and mild limitations in physical fitness include those of youngsters in the general population. Additional concerns relate to inability to sustain aerobic activity and musculoskeletal functioning within acceptable levels and incapacity for independent living and participation in daily living activities (including sport and movement activities).

Desired Profile

Boys and girls aged 10 to 17 years with intellectual disability and mild limitations in physical fitness should possess, at minimum, levels of aerobic behavior consistent with the ability to sustain moderate physical activity or progress toward a level of aerobic capacity consistent with positive health; body composition consistent with positive health; healthful levels of flexibility or range of motion (especially of the lower back); and levels of abdominal and upper-body strength and endurance appropriate for independent living, participation in physical activities, and progress toward performance levels of peers in the general population.

Components of Physical Fitness

Test items to assess aerobic functioning, body composition, and musculoskeletal functioning for this population appear in table 4.2.

HEALTH-RELATED, CRITERION-REFERENCED PHYSICAL FITNESS PARAMETERS

Table 4.2 Test-Item Selection Guide for Youngsters With Intellectual Disability and Mild Limitation in Physical Fitness

Fitness component	Test item	Selection guide
Aerobic functioning	SELECT ONE:	
	15 m PACER (aerobic capacity; ages 10–12) or 20 m PACER (aerobic capacity; ages 13–17)	R
	TAMT (aerobic behavior, level 1)	R
Body composition	SELECT ONE:	
	Percent body fat	R
	Skinfolds	
	Sum of triceps and calf	R
	Sum of triceps and subscapular	O
	Body mass index	O
Musculoskeletal functioning	SELECT ONE:	
	Dominant grip strength (ages 10–17)	O
	Isometric push-up (ages 10–12) or bench press (ages 13–17)	O
	SELECT ONE:	
	Extended-arm hang (ages 10–12)	R
	Flexed-arm hang (ages 13–17)	R
	SELECT ONE:	
	Back-saver sit-and-reach	R
	Shoulder stretch	O
	REQUIRED:	
	Modified curl-up	R
	Trunk lift	R

Abbreviations: R = recommended; O = optional.

Standards and Fitness Zones

The physical fitness of youngsters with intellectual disability is evaluated using both general and specific standards. Youngsters attaining HFZs based on general standards related to body composition, aerobic behavior, and flexibility meet acceptable health-related levels of physical fitness for the general population. Youngsters meeting AFZ levels based on specific standards for test items attain target levels of physical fitness adjusted for the effects of impairment. AFZ levels represent attainable steps in progressing toward acceptable levels of health-related physical fitness for the general population. Standards and fitness zones for youngsters with intellectual disability and mild limitation in fitness can be found in Fitness Zone tables 3 and 4, located at the end of the chapter.

Aerobic Functioning

Aerobic *capacity* in youngsters with intellectual disability is evaluated using AFZs and HFZs based on specific and general standards associated with the PACER. AFZs represent target levels of aerobic capacity adjusted for youngsters with intellectual disability. They reflect a 10 percent downward adjustment from the HFZ standards for $\dot{V}O_2$max recommended for youngsters in the general population. General standards and HFZs for $\dot{V}O_2$max represent levels of aerobic capacity consistent with minimizing potential risk for future health problems and with adequate functioning for daily living. Aerobic *behavior* is measured by the TAMT, in which performance for 15 minutes at level 1 is an HFZ based on a general standard representing ability to sustain moderate physical activity. The same standard exists for all levels of the test. Level 1 is the minimal test level recommended for youngsters with intellectual disability and mild limitations in physical fitness.

Body Composition

The HFZs based on general standards are recommended for evaluation of body composition of youngsters with intellectual disability and mild limitation in physical fitness. No adjustments are made for disability.

Musculoskeletal Functioning

HFZs and AFZs based on general and specific standards are used for evaluating dominant grip strength, extended-arm hang, isometric push-up, bench press, and flexed-arm hang for youngsters with intellectual disability and mild limitation in physical fitness. The AFZs reflect levels of strength or endurance adjusted for intellectual disability. Specific standards for youngsters with intellectual disability represent the following percentages of the performances of students in the general population: dominant grip strength, 65 percent; extended-arm hang, 75 percent; isometric push-up, bench press, flexed-arm hang, and modified curl-up, 50 percent.

Youngsters with intellectual disability can also be evaluated using general standards. For dominant grip, extended-arm hang, isometric push-up, and bench press, the general standards represent approximately the 20th percentile of performance by a Project Target sample of youth from the general population. General standards for flexed-arm hang and modified curl-up represent minimal standards for youth from the general population (Cooper Institute, 2013). It is recommended that HFZs based on general standards reflecting positive levels of physical fitness be used for evaluation of the back-saver sit-and-reach, trunk lift, and shoulder stretch.

Youngsters With Visual Impairment

Health-Related Concerns

Health-related needs and concerns of youngsters with visual impairment include those of students in the general population, as well as musculoskeletal functioning necessary for appropriate pelvic alignment and posture.

Desired Profile

Boys and girls aged 10 to 17 years should possess, at minimum, levels of maximal oxygen uptake and body composition consistent with positive health, flexibility for functional health (especially appropriate pelvic alignment and posture and functioning of the lower back), and levels of abdominal and upper-body strength and endurance adequate for independent living and participation in physical activities.

Components of Physical Fitness

Test items to assess aerobic functioning, body composition, and musculoskeletal functioning for this population appear in table 4.3.

Standards and Fitness Zones

Standards and fitness zones for youngsters with visual impairment (blindness) can be found in Fitness Zone tables 5 and 6, located at the end of the chapter.

HEALTH-RELATED, CRITERION-REFERENCED PHYSICAL FITNESS PARAMETERS

Table 4.3 Test-Item Selection Guide for Youngsters With Visual Impairment

Fitness component	Test item	Selection guide
Aerobic functioning	SELECT ONE:	
	PACER: 15 m or 20 m (aerobic capacity; ages 10–17)	R
	1-mile run/walk (aerobic capacity; ages 15–17)	O
	TAMT (aerobic behavior, level 1)	O
Body composition	SELECT ONE:	
	Percent body fat	R
	Skinfolds—sum of triceps and calf	R
	Body mass index	O
Musculoskeletal functioning	Required:	
	Curl-up	R
	Trunk lift	R
	SELECT ONE:	
	Push-up	R
	Pull-up	O
	Modified pull-up	O
	Flexed-arm hang	O
	SELECT ONE:	
	Back-saver sit-and-reach	R
	Shoulder stretch	O

Abbreviations: R = recommended; O = optional.

Aerobic Functioning

The HFZ standards used for evaluating aerobic functioning (aerobic capacity and aerobic behavior) for the general population can be used for youngsters with visual impairment. Specific standards are also available; those associated with the AFZ are recommended for youngsters who are blind and require assistance in performing the one-mile run/walk and the PACER. These specific standards are based on a 3 percent reduction of $\dot{V}O_2max$ standards associated with the general population. Remember, however, that most youngsters with visual impairment can be evaluated using the general standards that are used for their sighted peers.

Body Composition

The HFZs based on general standards for percentage body fat and BMI are recommended for youngsters with visual impairment. No adjustments are made for disability.

Musculoskeletal Functioning

It is recommended that youngsters with visual impairment be evaluated using HFZ levels based on general standards.

Youngsters With Spinal Cord Injury

Health-Related Concerns

Health-related needs and concerns typical of youngsters with spinal cord injury include those of students in the general population. Additional concerns include inability to sustain aerobic activity; lack of flexibility or range of motion in the hips and upper body, particularly the shoulder; lack of strength and endurance to lift and transfer the body independently, lift the body to prevent decubitus ulcers, and propel a wheelchair; and excessive body fat, which inhibits health.

Desired Profile

Individuals with spinal cord injury should possess, at minimum, the ability to sustain moderate physical activity, body composition consistent with positive health, levels of flexibility and range of motion to perform activities of daily living and to inhibit contractures, levels of muscular strength and endurance for wheelchair users to lift and transfer the body and push a wheelchair, muscular strength and endurance to counteract muscular weaknesses, and fitness levels needed to enhance the performance of daily living activities (including sport activities).

Components of Physical Fitness

Test items to assess aerobic functioning, body composition, and musculoskeletal functioning in this population appear in table 4.4.

Table 4.4 Test-Item Selection Guide for Youngsters With Spinal Cord Injury

Fitness component	Test item	Selection guide		
		LLQ Low-level (C6–C8) quadriplegic	SCI-PW Paraplegic- wheelchair	SCI-PA Paraplegic- ambulatory
Aerobic functioning	TAMT (aerobic behavior, level 1)	R	R	R
Body composition	SELECT ONE:			
	Percent body fat	R	R	R
	Skinfolds			
	Sum of triceps and subscapular	R	R	R
	Triceps only	O	O	O
Musculoskeletal functioning	REQUIRED (IF APPROPRIATE):			
	Seated push-up	O/TA[a]	R	
	SELECT ONE:			
	Reverse curl	R		
	Dominant grip strength		R	R
	Bench press (ages 13–17) or dumbbell press (dominant; ages 13–17)		O	O
	RECOMMENDED:			
	Modified Apley test		R	R
	Modified Thomas test			R
	TST[b]	R	R[c]	

Abbreviations: R = recommended; O = optional; TA = task analysis.

[a] Task analysis of test items for muscular strength and endurance or variations of test items that reflect the needs and abilities of the individual.

[b] Select at least two items from the TST on the basis of possible participant needs. For LLQ, shoulder abduction, shoulder external rotation, and forearm pronation are recommended. For SCI-PA, shoulder abduction and shoulder external rotation are recommended if the modified Apley test is not passed. Measure both extremities on the modified Apley, modified Thomas, and TST, and apply health-related standards as appropriate.

[c] Recommended if the modified Apley test is not passed with a score of 3.

HEALTH-RELATED, CRITERION-REFERENCED PHYSICAL FITNESS PARAMETERS

Standards and Fitness Zones

Standards and fitness zones recommended for the evaluation of youngsters with spinal cord injury appear in Fitness Zone tables 7 and 8, located at the end of the chapter.

Aerobic Functioning

For youngsters with spinal cord injury, aerobic behavior is measured using the TAMT. Completion of level 1 of the test for 15 minutes represents ability to sustain moderate physical activity and is the recommended HFZ for the test.

Body Composition

The HFZs based on general standards associated with percentage body fat are recommended for evaluating body composition; no adjustments are made for disability. The BMI test item is not recommended for youngsters with spinal cord injury.

Musculoskeletal Functioning

Musculoskeletal functioning is evaluated using a variety of standards in this population. General standards for HFZs for dominant grip strength, bench press, and dumbbell press are based on 20th percentile values of a sample of youngsters from the general population. The 5-second specific AFZ standard for the seated push-up is related to the recommendation that wheelchair users should relieve skin pressure on their buttocks and legs for at least 5 seconds every 15 minutes. The 20-second standard is a higher level of strength and endurance that enhances lifting and transferring of the body, as well as wheelchair propulsion.

The AFZ based on the specific standard for the reverse curl is tied directly to the functional ability to lift a 1-pound (0.5-kilogram) weight one time. The HFZs based on general standards for the modified Apley and Thomas tests (a score of 3) indicate, respectively, that youngsters have optimal flexibility of the shoulder joint and optimal hip extension. A score of 1 on target stretch test (TST) items indicates a functional range of motion in a joint associated with the AFZ. A score of 2 is the HFZ, reflecting optimal flexibility in a joint.

Youngsters With Cerebral Palsy

Health-Related Concerns

Health-related needs and concerns of youngsters with cerebral palsy include those typical for students in the general population. Additional concerns include inability to sustain aerobic activity; lack of flexibility or range of motion in various joints of the body; insufficient muscular strength and endurance to maintain muscular balance and body symmetry; inability to engage in independent mobility, lift and transfer the body, perform activities of daily living, and participate in leisure activities; and either excessive or insufficient body fat, which inhibits health.

Desired Profile

Individuals with cerebral palsy should possess, at minimum, the ability to sustain moderate physical activity; body composition consistent with positive health; and levels of flexibility and muscular strength and endurance to foster independent living (including mobility), muscle balance and body symmetry, and participation in a variety of physical activities (including sport or leisure activities).

Components of Physical Fitness

Test items to assess aerobic functioning, body composition, and musculoskeletal functioning in this population appear in table 4.5.

Standards and Fitness Zones

Standards recommended for evaluation pertain only to test items designated as recommended or optional for youngsters with cerebral palsy. Musculoskeletal functioning standards may be associated with specific classifications. Youngsters with cerebral palsy are required to attain standards on only one side of the body (i.e., dominant or preferred side) for the following items: modified Apley test, TST, dumbbell press, and dominant grip strength. Standards and fitness zones for youngsters with cerebral palsy can be found in Fitness Zone tables 9 and 10, located at the end of the chapter.

Aerobic Functioning

For youngsters with cerebral palsy, aerobic behavior is measured using the TAMT. Completion of level 1 of the test for 15 minutes represents the ability to sustain moderate physical activity and is the recommended HFZ based on a general standard.

Body Composition

An HFZ based on general standards for percentage body fat is recommended for youngsters with cerebral palsy; no adjustment is made for disability. HFZs represent optimal levels of body fat. Skinfold measures and body mass index relate to these body fat ranges; BMI should be used only if height and weight can be measured accurately.

Musculoskeletal Functioning

Musculoskeletal functioning is evaluated using a variety of standards. HFZs based on general standards for dominant grip and dumbbell press are based on 20th percentile values of a sample of youngsters from the general population. The standard for the 40-meter push/walk is suggested for functional mobility, which reflects a level of musculoskeletal ability involving strength, endurance, and flexibility. The 5-second specific standard for the seated push-up is related to the recommendation that wheelchair users should relieve the skin pressure on their buttocks and legs for at least 5 seconds every 15 minutes. The 20-second specific standard represents a higher level of strength and endurance, which enhances muscular balance around the elbow, ability to transfer the body, and ability to propel a wheelchair.

The 8-foot (2.4-meter) specific standard for the wheelchair ramp test reflects the ability to ascend a ramp with approximately one step of elevation (8 inches or 20 centimeters), such as would be found at a corner curb cut. The 15-foot (4.6-meter) specific standard in the AFZ can vary (at the discretion of the tester) as a function of the length of a ramp that a specific young person might frequently encounter in his or her environment.

HEALTH-RELATED, CRITERION-REFERENCED PHYSICAL FITNESS PARAMETERS

HEALTH-RELATED, CRITERION-REFERENCED PHYSICAL FITNESS PARAMETERS

Table 4.5 Test-Item Selection Guide for Youngsters With Cerebral Palsy

Fitness component	Test item	Selection guide								
		CPISRA sport classifications								
		Motorized wheelchair	Wheelchair					Ambulatory		
		C1[a]	C2U[b]	C2L[b]	C3	C4	C5	C6	C7	C8
Aerobic functioning	TAMT (aerobic behavior, level 1)	R	R	R	R	R	R	R	R	R
Body composition	**SELECT ONE:**									
	Percent body fat	R	R	R	R	R	R	R	R	R
	Skinfolds									
	Sum of triceps and subscapular	R	R	R	R	R	R	R	R	R
	Triceps only	O	O	O	O	O	O	O	O	O
	Body mass index	O	O	O	O	O	O	O	O	O
Musculoskeletal functioning	**SELECT ONE OR MORE:**									
	Modified Apley test[c,d]	R	R		R	R	R	R	R	R
	Modified Thomas test[c]						R	R	R	R
	TST[e]	R	R	R	R	R	O	O	O	O
	SELECT ONE OR MORE (EXCEPT FOR C1):[a]									
	Seated push-up[f]		R		R	R		R		
	40 m wheelchair push		R	R	O					
	40 m walk							R		
	Dominant grip strength					O	O		O	O
	Dumbbell press (dominant; ages 13–17)				O	O	O		R	R
	Wheelchair ramp test				R					

Abbreviations: R = recommended; O = optional.

[a] If recommended test items are inappropriate for individuals classified as C1, it is recommended that these test items or alternatives important to the individual be task-analyzed and used in connection with individual developmental progress.

[b] C2 participants with a higher degree of functioning in the upper extremities are classified 2U, and those with a higher degree of functioning in the lower extremities are classified as 2L.

[c] Test one or both extremities, as possible.

[d] Omit this item for C1 subjects using assistive devices.

[e] Test items should be administered on right and left extremities, as appropriate. TST items particularly important for people with cerebral palsy include elbow and shoulder extension, shoulder abduction, shoulder external rotation, and forearm supination. For ambulatory people, knee extension measurements may be particularly important.

[f] Test item is not recommended for hemiplegic C3 and C4 participants. Hemiplegic participants should be given the dumbbell press.

Standards for the modified Apley test, modified Thomas test, and TST vary for each classification. Modified Apley test standards are derived on a logical basis (see chapter 2 for description). The general standard for HFZ for the modified Apley test (a score of 3) is recommended for youngsters in classes C2U to C8. An AFZ based on a specific standard of 2 is recommended for classes C1 and C2L. Modified Thomas test standards relate to flexibility of the hip flexors. An AFZ based on a general standard for the modified Thomas test (a score of 3) is recommended for youngsters in classes C6 and C8. An AFZ based on a specific standard of 2 is recommended for class C5. For class C7 (hemiplegia), a score of 3 is recommended for the unaffected side of the body, and a score of 2 is recommended for the affected side. The TST standard for youngsters in most classes (C3 through C8) is a score of 1, which represents a clinically accepted functional range of motion in a joint. An HFZ based on a general standard (a score of 2) represents optimal range of motion for a particular joint. The TST is also recommended for classes C1 and C2; however, individualized standards are recommended for these classes. Standards for the TST and modified Apley test for youngsters with cerebral palsy are applied to the dominant or preferred side of the body.

Youngsters With Congenital Anomaly or Amputation

Health-Related Concerns

Health-related needs and concerns of youngsters with congenital anomaly or amputation include those typical of students in the general population. Additional concerns include inability to sustain aerobic activity; lack of upper- and lower-body flexibility or range of motion; lack of muscular strength and endurance of wheelchair users to lift and transfer the body independently; inability to overcome architectural barriers, lift the body to prevent decubitus ulcers, and propel a wheelchair; and excessive body fat, which inhibits health.

Desired Profile

Individuals with congenital anomaly or amputation should possess, at minimum and as appropriate, the ability to sustain moderate physical activity or physical activity that promotes levels of functioning consistent with positive health; body composition consistent with positive health; levels of flexibility and range of motion to perform activities of daily living and inhibit contractures; levels of muscular strength and endurance in wheelchair users to lift and transfer the body, overcome architectural barriers, and propel a wheelchair; abdominal and upper-body muscular strength and endurance to counteract muscular weakness; and fitness levels needed to enhance performance of daily living activities (including sport and movement activities).

Components of Physical Fitness

Test items to assess aerobic functioning, body composition, and musculoskeletal functioning in this population appear in table 4.6.

HEALTH-RELATED, CRITERION-REFERENCED PHYSICAL FITNESS PARAMETERS

Table 4.6 Test-Item Selection Guide for Youngsters With Congenital Anomaly or Amputation

Fitness component	Test item	Selection guide / Subclassification					
		One arm only	Two arms only	One leg only	Two legs only	One arm, one leg (same side)	One arm, one leg (opposite side)
Aerobic functioning	**SELECT ONE:**						
	PACER: 15 m, 20 m (ages 10–17; aerobic capacity)	R	R				
	1-mile run/walk (aerobic capacity)	O	O				
	TAMT (aerobic behavior, level 1)			R	R	R	R
Body composition	**SELECT ONE:**						
	Percent body fat	R	R	R	R	R	R
	Skinfolds						
	Triceps only	R	R[a]	R	R	R	R
	Sum of triceps and subscapular	O	O[a]	R	R	R	R
	Sum of triceps and calf	R	O[a]	O		O	O
Musculoskeletal functioning	**SELECT ONE (UNAFFECTED LIMB[S]):**						
	Shoulder stretch or modified Apley test	R		R	R	R	R
	Back-saver sit-and-reach	R		R		R	
	SELECT AS NEEDED (AFFECTED LIMBS); TST[b]:						
	Knee extension			O[c,d,e]	O[c,d,e]	O[c,d,e]	O[c,d,e]
	Shoulder flexion	O[d,e]	O[d,e]			O[d,e]	O[d,e]
	External shoulder rotation	O[d,e]	O[d,e]			O[d,e]	O[d,e]
	Elbow extension	O[d,e]	O[d,e]			R[d,e]	R[d,e]
	REQUIRED:						
	Trunk lift	R	R				
	Curl-up	R	R				
	SELECT ONE:						
	Dumbbell press (dominant; ages 13–17)	R		O	O	R	R
	Bench press (ages 13–17)			R	R		
	Seated push-up			R[f]	R[f]		
	Dominant grip strength	O		O	O	O	O

[a] Selection depends on site of anomaly or amputation.

[b] If additional unique range-of-motion needs are suspected, relevant joints may be tested using the TST.

[c] Optional for below-knee amputation or anomaly of affected limbs only.

[d] Optional in cases where measurement is possible and appropriate.

[e] If potential is not limited by impairment, target scores of 1 or above on the TST are attainable. If impairment affects extent of movement, the TST may be used to obtain scores from which to determine individual status and progress.

[f] Recommended only for wheelchair users.

Standards and Fitness Zones

Standards and fitness zones recommended for evaluation of youngsters with congenital anomaly or amputation can be found in Fitness Zone tables 11 and 12, located at the end of the chapter.

Aerobic Functioning

Aerobic behavior is measured using the TAMT. Completion of level 1 of the test for 15 minutes represents ability to sustain moderate physical activity and is the recommended general standard for the test. General standards for aerobic capacity (via the PACER and one-mile run/walk) are also provided, but test users are cautioned that results will likely be affected by loss of limb or function (especially for the one-mile run/walk).

Body Composition

HFZ levels based on general standards are used for skinfolds tied to percentage body fat; no adjustment is made for disability. BMI is not recommended for youngsters with congenital anomaly or amputation.

Musculoskeletal Functioning

Musculoskeletal functioning is evaluated using a variety of standards. HFZs based on general standards for dominant grip strength, dumbbell press, and bench press are based on 20th percentile values of the Project Target (1998) sample of youth from the general population. HFZ levels based on general standards for the curl-up *and* trunk lift correspond to values associated with Fitnessgram standards for youth in the general population (Cooper Institute, 2013). For subclassifications of people for whom the shoulder stretch, back-saver sit-and-reach, and modified Apley test are recommended for unaffected limbs, general standards are recommended for evaluation. Standards for these items reflect acceptable levels of flexibility. As indicated in table 4.6, selected items on the TST are recommended for various subclassifications. If potential is not limited by an impairment, a target score of 1 or above should be attainable. If an impairment affects extent of movement, the TST may be used to obtain scores for use in determining an individual's present status and progress. A score of 1 is the specific standard associated with an AFZ reflecting functional range of motion, and a score of 2 is the general standard associated with an HFZ reflecting optimal range of motion.

HEALTH-RELATED, CRITERION-REFERENCED PHYSICAL FITNESS PARAMETERS

Fitness Zone Tables
for Recommended and Optional Test Items

This section provides the fitness zones that can be used with various populations of youngsters with disabilities. Fitness Zone tables 3 through 12 are available for printing from the web resource at www.HumanKinetics.com/BrockportPhysicalFitnessTestManual by using the pass code Brockport58743AR7.

Fitness Zone Table 1   Boys' Fitnessgram Standards for Healthy Fitness Zone

Age (yr.)	Aerobic capacity $\dot{V}O_2MAX$ (ml/kg/min.) PACER, 1-mile run, and walk test			Percent body fat				Body mass index			
	NI-Health risk*	NI	HFZ	Very lean	HFZ	NI	NI—health risk	Very lean	HFZ	NI	NI—health risk
5	Completion of test. Lap count or time standards not recommended.			≤8.8	8.9–18.8	18.9	≥27.0	≤13.8	13.9–16.8	16.9	≥18.1
6				≤8.4	8.5–18.8	18.9	≥27.0	≤13.7	13.8–17.1	17.2	≥18.8
7				≤8.2	8.3–18.8	18.9	≥27.0	≤13.7	13.8–17.6	17.7	≥19.6
8				≤8.3	8.4–18.8	18.9	≥27.0	≤13.9	14.0–18.2	18.3	≥20.6
9				≤8.6	8.7–20.6	20.7	≥30.1	≤14.1	14.2–18.9	19.0	≥21.6
10	≤37.3	37.4–40.1	≥40.2	≤8.8	8.9–22.4	22.5	≥33.2	≤14.4	14.5–19.7	19.8	≥22.7
11	≤37.3	37.4–40.1	≥40.2	≤8.7	8.8–23.6	23.7	≥35.4	≤14.8	14.9–20.5	20.6	≥23.7
12	≤37.6	37.7–40.2	≥40.3	≤8.3	8.4–23.6	23.7	≥35.9	≤15.2	15.3–21.3	21.4	≥24.7
13	≤38.6	38.7–41.0	≥41.1	≤7.7	7.8–22.8	22.9	≥35.0	≤15.7	15.8–22.2	22.3	≥25.6
14	≤39.6	39.7–42.4	≥42.5	≤7.0	7.1–21.3	21.4	≥33.2	≤16.3	16.4–23.0	23.1	≥26.5
15	≤40.6	40.7–43.5	≥43.6	≤6.5	6.6–20.1	20.2	≥31.5	≤16.8	16.9–23.7	23.8	≥27.2
16	≤41.0	41.1–44.0	≥44.1	≤6.4	6.5–20.1	20.2	≥31.6	≤17.4	17.5–24.5	24.6	≥27.9
17	≤41.2	41.3–44.1	≥44.2	≤6.6	6.7–20.9	21.0	≥33.0	≤18.0	18.1–24.9	25.0	≥28.6
>17	≤41.2	41.3–44.2	≥44.3	≤6.9	7.0–22.2	22.3	≥35.1	≤18.5	18.6–24.9	25.0	≥29.3

Age (yr.)	Curl-up (no. completed)	Trunk lift (in.)	90° push-up (no. completed)	Modified pull-up (no. completed)	Flexed-arm hang (sec.)	Back-saver sit-and-reach† (in.)	Shoulder stretch
5	≥2	6–12	≥3	≥2	≥2	8	Healthy Fitness Zone = touching fingertips together behind the back on both the right and left sides.
6	≥2	6–12	≥3	≥2	≥2	8	
7	≥4	6–12	≥4	≥3	≥3	8	
8	≥6	6–12	≥5	≥4	≥3	8	
9	≥9	6–12	≥6	≥5	≥4	8	
10	≥12	9–12	≥7	≥5	≥4	8	
11	≥15	9–12	≥8	≥6	≥6	8	
12	≥18	9–12	≥10	≥7	≥10	8	
13	≥21	9–12	≥12	≥8	≥12	8	
14	≥24	9–12	≥14	≥9	≥15	8	
15	≥24	9–12	≥16	≥10	≥15	8	
16	≥24	9–12	≥18	≥12	≥15	8	
17	≥24	9–12	≥18	≥14	≥15	8	
>17	≥24	9–12	≥18	≥14	≥15	8	

Age	PACER (20m laps)		
	NI HR[a]	NI[a]	HFZ[b]
5–9	Completion of test. Lap count or time standards not recommended.		
10	8	9–16	≥17
11	11	12–19	≥20
12	15	16–22	≥23
13	21	22–28	≥29
14	27	28–35	≥36
15	33	34–41	≥42
16	37	38–46	≥47
17	41	42–49	≥50

*NI = Needs improvement.

†Test is scored yes/no; must reach this distance on each side to achieve the HFZ.

Reprinted, by permission, from The Cooper Institute, 2013, *Fitnessgram/Activitygram test administration manual*, updated 4th ed. (Champaign, IL: Human Kinetics), 65.

[a]NI HR and NI lap counts from Winnick and Short, 2014, developed with an equation provided by The Cooper Institute (2013).

[b]Reprinted, by permission, from The Cooper Institute, 2014, *Goal setting chart for aerobic capacity and PACER test*.

Fitness Zone Table 2 Girls' Fitnessgram Standards for Healthy Fitness Zone

Age (yr.)	Aerobic capacity V̇O₂MAX (ml/kg/min.) PACER, 1-mile run, and walk test			Percent body fat				Body mass index			
	NI-Health risk*	NI	HFZ	Very lean	HFZ	NI	NI— health risk	Very lean	HFZ	NI	NI— health risk
5	Completion of test. Lap count or time standards not recommended.			≤9.7	9.8–20.8	20.9	≥28.4	≤13.5	13.6–16.8	16.9	≥18.5
6				≤9.8	9.9–20.8	20.9	≥28.4	≤13.4	13.5–17.0	17.3	≥19.2
7				≤10.0	10.1–20.8	20.9	≥28.4	≤13.5	13.5–17.5	18.0	≥20.2
8				≤10.4	20.5–20.8	20.9	≥28.4	≤13.6	13.6–18.2	18.7	≥21.2
9				≤10.9	11.0–22.6	22.7	≥30.8	≤13.9	13.8–18.9	19.5	≥22.4
10	≤37.3	37.4–40.1	≥40.2	≤11.5	11.6–24.3	24.4	≥33.0	≤14.2	14.3–20.3	20.4	≥23.6
11	≤37.3	37.4–40.1	≥40.2	≤12.1	12.2–25.7	25.8	≥34.5	≤14.6	14.7–21.2	21.3	≥24.7
12	≤37.0	37.1–40.0	≥40.1	≤12.6	12.7–26.7	26.8	≥35.5	≤15.1	15.2–22.1	22.2	≥25.8
13	≤36.6	68.7–39.6	≥39.7	≤13.3	13.4–27.7	27.8	≥36.3	≤15.6	15.7–22.9	23.0	≥26.8
14	≤36.3	36.4–39.3	≥39.4	≤13.9	14.0–28.5	28.6	≥36.8	≤16.1	16.2–23.6	23.7	≥27.7
15	36.0	36.1–39.0	≥39.1	≤14.5	14.6–29.1	29.2	≥37.1	≤16.6	16.7–24.3	24.4	≥28.5
16	≤35.8	35.9–38.8	≥38.9	≤15.2	15.3–29.7	29.8	≥37.4	≤17.0	17.1–24.8	24.9	≥29.3
17	≤35.7	35.8–38.7	≥38.8	≤15.8	15.9–30.4	20.5	≥37.9	≤17.4	17.5–24.9	25.0	≥30.0
>17	≤35.3	35.4–38.5	≥38.6	≤16.4	16.5–31.3	31.4	≥38.6	≤17.7	17.8–24.9	25.0	≥30.0

Age (yr.)	Curl-up (no. completed)	Trunk lift (in.)	90° push-up (no. completed)	Modified pull-up (no. completed)	Flexed-arm hang (sec.)	Back-saver sit-and-reach† (in.)	Shoulder stretch
5	≥2	6–12	≥3	≥2	≥2	9	Healthy Fitness Zone = touching fingertips together behind the back on both the right and left sides.
6	≥2	6–12	≥3	≥2	≥2	9	
7	≥4	6–12	≥4	≥3	≥3	9	
8	≥6	6–12	≥5	≥4	≥3	9	
9	≥9	6–12	≥6	≥4	≥4	9	
10	≥12	9–12	≥7	≥4	≥4	9	
11	≥15	9–12	≥7	≥4	≥6	10	
12	≥18	9–12	≥7	≥4	≥7	10	
13	≥18	9–12	≥7	≥4	≥8	10	
14	≥18	9–12	≥7	≥4	≥8	10	
15	≥18	9–12	≥7	≥4	≥8	12	
16	≥18	9–12	≥7	≥4	≥8	12	
17	≥18	9–12	≥7	≥4	≥8	12	
>17	≥18	9–12	≥7	≥4	≥8	12	

Age	PACER (20m laps)		
	NI HRᵃ	NIᵃ	HFZᵇ
5–9	Completion of test. Lap count or time standards not recommended.		
10	8	9–16	≥17
11	11	12–19	≥20
12	13	14–22	≥23
13	15	16–24	≥25
14	17	18–26	≥27
15	20	21–29	≥30
16	22	23–31	≥32
17	25	26–34	≥35

*NI = Needs improvement.

†Test is scored yes/no; must reach this distance on each side to achieve the HFZ.

Reprinted, by permission, from The Cooper Institute, 2013, *Fitnessgram/Activitygram test administration manual*, updated 4th ed. (Champaign, IL: Human Kinetics), 66.

ᵃNI HR and NI lap counts from Winnick and Short, 2014, developed with an equation provided by The Cooper Institute (2013).

ᵇReprinted, by permission, from The Cooper Institute, 2014, *Goal setting chart for aerobic capacity and PACER test.*

Fitness Zone Table 3   Boys With Intellectual Disability

Age (yr.)	PACER (20 m laps)			TAMT (pass/fail)		Percent body fat[c]				Triceps and calf skinfold[e] (mm)		Body mass index[c]			
	NI[a]	AFZ[a]	HFZ[b]	HFZ[d]	NI	Very lean	HFZ	NI	NI (health risk)	HFZ	NI (health risk)	Very lean	HFZ	NI	NI (health risk)
10	≤4	5–16	≥17	P	F	≤8.8	8.9–22.4	22.5	≥33.2	11–29	≥33.2	≤14.4	14.5–19.7	19.8	≥22.7
11	≤7	8–19	≥20	P	F	≤8.7	8.8–23.6	23.7	≥35.4	11–31	≥35.4	≤14.8	14.9–20.5	20.6	≥23.7
12	≤11	12–22	≥23	P	F	≤8.3	8.4–23.6	23.7	≥35.9	10–31	≥35.9	≤15.2	15.3–21.3	21.4	≥24.7
13	≤16	17–28	≥29	P	F	≤7.7	7.8–22.8	22.9	≥35.0	9–30	≥35.0	≤15.7	15.8–22.2	22.3	≥25.6
14	≤23	24–35	≥36	P	F	≤7.0	7.1–21.3	21.4	≥33.2	8–28	≥33.2	≤16.3	16.4–23.0	23.1	≥26.5
15	≤29	30–41	≥42	P	F	≤6.5	6.6–20.1	20.2	≥31.5	8–26	≥31.5	≤16.8	16.9–23.7	23.8	≥27.2
16	≤33	34–46	≥47	P	F	≤6.4	6.5–20.1	20.2	≥31.6	8–26	≥31.6	≤17.4	17.5–24.5	24.6	≥27.9
17	≤37	38–49	≥50	P	F	≤6.6	6.7–20.9	21.0	≥33.0	8–27	≥33.0	≤18.0	18.1–24.9	25.0	≥28.6

Age (yr.)	Isometric push-up (sec.)			Bench press (# completed)			Extended-arm hang (sec.)			Flexed-arm hang (sec.)			Grip strength (kg)			Modified curl-up (# completed)		
	NI	AFZ	HFZ[d]	NI	AFZ	HFZ[d]	NI	AFZ	HFZ[d]	NI	AFZ	HFZ[c]	NI	AFZ	HFZ[d]	NI	AFZ	HFZ[c]
10	≤19	20–39	40				≤22	23–29	30–40				≤11	12–17	≥18	≤6	7–11	≥12
11	≤19	20–39	40				≤22	23–29	30–40				≤13	14–20	≥21	≤8	9–14	≥15
12	≤19	20–39	40				≤22	23–29	30–40				≤15	16–24	≥25	≤10	11–17	≥18
13				≤9	10–19	20–50				≤5	6–11	≥12	≤18	19–28	≥29	≤12	13–20	≥21
14				≤15	16–32	33–50				≤7	8–14	≥15	≤21	22–32	≥33	≤13	14–23	≥24
15				≤19	20–39	40–50				≤7	8–14	≥15	≤23	24–36	≥37	≤13	14–23	≥24
16				≤22	23–46	47–50				≤7	8–14	≥15	≤27	28–42	≥43	≤13	14–23	≥24
17				≤24	25–49	50				≤7	8–14	≥15	≤31	32–48	≥49	≤13	14–23	≥24

Age (yr.)	Trunk lift (in.)		Shoulder stretch (pass/fail)		Sit-and-reach (in.)	
	NI	HFZ[c]	NI	HFZ[c]	NI	HFZ[c]
10	≤8	9–12	F	P	≤7	8
11	≤8	9–12	F	P	≤7	8
12	≤8	9–12	F	P	≤7	8
13	≤8	9–12	F	P	≤7	8
14	≤8	9–12	F	P	≤7	8
15	≤8	9–12	F	P	≤7	8
16	≤8	9–12	F	P	≤7	8
17	≤8	9–12	F	P	≤7	8

a. NI and AFZ lap counts from Winnick and Short, 2014, developed with an equation provided by The Cooper Institute (2013). AFZ lap range represents a 10 percent reduction from $\dot{V}O_2$max standard for the general population. Where appropriate, youngsters with intellectual disability should pursue standards for the HFZ.

b. Reprinted, by permission, from The Cooper Institute, 2014, Goal setting chart for aerobic capacity and PACER test.

c. Reprinted, by permission, from The Cooper Institute, 2013, Fitnessgram/Activitygram test administration manual, updated 4th ed. (Champaign, IL: Human Kinetics), 65.

d. Based on Project Target (1998).

e. The Cooper Institute, 2013, Fitnessgram/Activitygram test administration manual, updated 4th ed. (Champaign, IL: Human Kinetics), 65, 101.

Fitness Zone Table 4 Girls With Intellectual Disability

Age (yr.)	PACER (20 m laps)			TAMT (pass/fail)		Percent body fat				Triceps and calf skinfold[e] (mm)			Body mass index[c]		
	NI[a]	AFZ[a]	HFZ[b]	NI	HFZ[d]	Very lean	HFZ	NI	NI (health risk)	Very lean	HFZ	NI (health risk)	HFZ	NI	NI (health risk)
10	≤4	5–16	≥17	F	P	≤11.5	11.6–24.3	24.4	≥33.0	≤14.2	11–32	≥23.6	14.3–20.3	20.4	≥23.6
11	≤7	8–19	≥20	F	P	≤12.1	12.2–25.7	25.8	≥34.5	≤14.6	12–34	≥24.7	14.7–21.2	21.3	≥24.7
12	≤10	11–22	≥23	F	P	≤12.6	12.7–26.7	26.8	≥35.5	≤15.1	13–36	≥25.8	15.2–22.1	22.2	≥25.8
13	≤12	13–24	≥25	F	P	≤13.3	13.4–27.7	27.8	≥36.3	≤15.6	14–37	≥26.8	15.7–22.9	23.0	≥26.8
14	≤15	16–26	≥27	F	P	≤13.9	14.0–28.5	28.6	≥36.8	≤16.1	15–39	≥27.7	16.2–23.6	23.7	≥27.7
15	≤17	18–29	≥30	F	P	≤14.5	14.6–29.1	29.2	≥37.1	≤16.6	16–40	≥28.5	16.7–24.3	24.4	≥28.5
16	≤20	21–31	≥32	F	P	≤15.2	15.3–29.7	29.8	≥37.4	≤17.0	17–41	≥29.3	17.1–24.8	24.9	≥29.3
17	≤23	24–34	≥35	F	P	≤15.8	15.9–30.4	30.5	≥37.9	≤17.4	18–42	≥30.0	17.5–24.9	25.0	≥30.0

Age (yr.)	Isometric push-up (sec.)			Bench press (# completed)			Extended-arm hang (sec.)			Flexed-arm hang (sec.)			Grip strength (kg)			Modified curl-up (# completed)		
	NI	AFZ	HFZ[d]	NI	AFZ	HFZ[d]	NI	AFZ	HFZ[d]	NI	AFZ	HFZ[c]	NI	AFZ	HFZ[d]	NI	AFZ	HFZ[c]
10	≤12	13–24	25–40				≤14	15–19	20–40				≤10	11–16	≥17	≤6	7–11	≥12
11	≤12	13–24	25–40				≤14	15–19	20–40				≤11	12–18	≥19	≤8	9–14	≥15
12	≤12	13–24	25–40				≤14	15–19	20–40				≤13	14–21	≥22	≤10	11–17	≥18
13				≤4	5–9	10–50				≤3	4–7	≥8	≤15	16–23	≥24	≤10	11–17	≥18
14				≤5	6–12	13–50				≤3	4–7	≥8	≤16	17–25	≥26	≤10	11–17	≥18
15				≤6	7–13	14–50				≤3	4–7	≥8	≤18	19–28	≥29	≤10	11–17	≥18
16				≤6	7–13	14–50				≤3	4–7	≥8	≤18	19–28	≥29	≤10	11–17	≥18
17				≤7	8–14	15–50				≤3	4–7	≥8	≤18	19–28	≥29	≤10	11–17	≥18

Age (yr.)	Trunk lift (in.)		Shoulder stretch (pass/fail)		Sit-and-reach (in.)	
	NI	HFZ[c]	NI	HFZ[c]	NI	HFZ[c]
10	≤8	9–12	F	P	≤8	9
11	≤8	9–12	F	P	≤9	10
12	≤8	9–12	F	P	≤9	10
13	≤8	9–12	F	P	≤9	10
14	≤8	9–12	F	P	≤9	10
15	≤8	9–12	F	P	≤11	12
16	≤8	9–12	F	P	≤11	12
17	≤8	9–12	F	P	≤11	12

a. NI and AFZ lap counts from Winnick and Short, 2014, developed with an equation provided by The Cooper Institute (2013). AFZ lap range represents a 10 percent reduction from $\dot{V}O_2$max standard for the general population. Where appropriate, youngsters with intellectual disability should pursue standards for the HFZ.

b. Reprinted, by permission, from The Cooper Institute, 2014, Goal setting chart for aerobic capacity and PACER test.

c. Reprinted, by permission, from The Cooper Institute, 2013, Fitnessgram/Activitygram test administration manual, updated 4th ed. (Champaign, IL: Human Kinetics), 66.

d. Based on data from Project Target (1998).

e. The Cooper Institute, 2013, Fitnessgram/Activitygram test administration manual, updated 4th ed. (Champaign, IL: Human Kinetics), 66, 102.

Fitness Zone Table 5   Boys With Visual Impairment (Blindness)

Age (yr.)	PACER (20 m laps) NI[a]	PACER AFZ[a]	PACER HFZ[b]	1-mile run (VO₂MAX) NI	1-mile run AFZ[a]	1-mile run HFZ[c]	TAMT (pass/fail) NI	TAMT HFZ[d]	Percent body fat[c] Very lean	Percent body fat HFZ	Percent body fat NI	Percent body fat NI (health risk)	Triceps and calf skinfold[f] (mm) HFZ
10	≤12	13–16	≥17	≤38.9	39.0–40.1	≥40.2	F	P	≤8.8	8.9–22.4	22.5	≥33.2	11–29
11	≤15	16–19	≥20	≤38.9	39.0–40.1	≥40.2	F	P	≤8.7	8.8–23.6	23.7	≥35.4	11–31
12	≤19	20–22	≥23	≤39.0	39.1–40.2	≥40.3	F	P	≤8.3	8.4–23.6	23.7	≥35.9	10–31
13	≤24	25–28	≥29	≤39.8	39.9–41.0	≥41.1	F	P	≤7.7	7.8–22.8	22.9	≥35.0	9–30
14	≤31	32–35	≥36	≤41.1	41.2–42.4	≥42.5	F	P	≤7.0	7.1–21.3	21.4	≥33.2	8–28
15	≤37	38–41	≥42	≤42.2	42.3–43.5	≥43.6	F	P	≤6.5	6.6–20.1	20.2	≥31.5	8–26
16	≤42	43–46	≥47	≤42.7	42.8–44.0	≥44.1	F	P	≤6.4	6.5–20.1	20.2	≥31.6	8–26
17	≤45	46–49	≥50	≤42.8	42.9–44.1	≥44.2	F	P	≤6.6	6.7–20.9	21.0	≥33.0	8–27

Age (yr.)	Body mass index[c] Very lean	BMI HFZ	BMI NI	BMI NI (health risk)	Flexed-arm hang (sec.) NI	Flexed-arm hang HFZ[c]	Push-up (# completed) NI	Push-up HFZ[c]	Pull-up (# completed) NI	Pull-up HFZ[e]	Modified pull-up (# completed) NI	Modified pull-up HFZ[c]	Curl-up (# completed) NI	Curl-up HFZ[c]
10	14.4	14.5–19.7	19.8	≥22.7	≤3	≥4	≤6	≥7	0	≥1	≤4	≥5	≤11	≥12
11	14.8	14.9–20.5	20.6	≥23.7	≤5	≥6	≤7	≥8	0	≥1	≤5	≥6	≤14	≥15
12	15.2	15.3–21.3	21.4	≥24.7	≤9	≥10	≤9	≥10	0	≥1	≤6	≥7	≤17	≥18
13	15.7	15.8–22.2	22.3	≥25.6	≤11	≥12	≤11	≥12	0	≥1	≤7	≥8	≤20	≥21
14	16.3	16.4–23.0	23.1	≥26.5	≤14	≥15	≤13	≥14	≤1	≥2	≤8	≥9	≤23	≥24
15	16.8	16.9–23.7	23.8	≥27.2	≤14	≥15	≤15	≥16	≤2	≥3	≤9	≥10	≤23	≥24
16	17.4	17.5–24.5	24.6	≥27.9	≤14	≥15	≤17	≥18	≤4	≥5	≤11	≥12	≤23	≥24
17	18.0	18.1–24.9	25.0	≥28.6	≤14	≥15	≤17	≥18	≤4	≥5	≤13	≥14	≤23	≥24

Age (yr.)	Trunk lift (in.) NI	Trunk lift HFZ[c]	Shoulder stretch (pass/fail) NI	Shoulder stretch HFZ[c]	Sit-and-reach (in.) NI	Sit-and-reach HFZ[c]
10	≤8	9–12	F	P	≤7	8
11	≤8	9–12	F	P	≤7	8
12	≤8	9–12	F	P	≤7	8
13	≤8	9–12	F	P	≤7	8
14	≤8	9–12	F	P	≤7	8
15	≤8	9–12	F	P	≤7	8
16	≤8	9–12	F	P	≤7	8
17	≤8	9–12	F	P	≤7	8

a. NI and AFZ lap counts from Winnick and Short, 2014, developed with an equation provided by The Cooper Institute (2013). AFZ lap range represents a 3 percent reduction from V̇O₂max standard for the general population. Where appropriate, youngsters with visual impairment should pursue standards for the HFZ.

b. Reprinted, by permission, from The Cooper Institute, 2014, *Goal setting chart for aerobic capacity and PACER test*.

c. Reprinted, by permission, from The Cooper Institute, 2013, *Fitnessgram/Activitygram test administration manual*, updated 4th ed. (Champaign, IL: Human Kinetics), 61.

d. Based on data from Project Target (1998).

e. Based on data from The Cooper Institute (1999).

f. The Cooper Institute, 2013, *Fitnessgram/Activitygram test administration manual*, updated 4th ed. (Champaign, IL: Human Kinetics), 65, 101.

Fitness Zone Table 6 Girls With Visual Impairment (Blindness)

Age (yr.)	PACER (20 m laps)			1-mile run (VO₂MAX)			TAMT (pass/fail)		Percent body fat				Triceps and calf skinfold[f] (mm)
	NI[a]	AFZ[a]	HFZ[b]	NI	AFZ[a]	HFZ[c]	NI	HFZ[d]	>Very lean	HFZ	NI	NI (health risk)	HFZ
10	≤12	13-16	≥17	≤38.9	39.0-40.1	≥40.2	F	P	≤11.5	11.6-24.3	24.4	≥33.0	11-32
11	≤15	16-19	≥20	≤38.9	39.0-40.1	≥40.2	F	P	≤12.1	12.2-25.7	25.8	≥34.5	12-34
12	≤18	19-22	≥23	≤38.8	38.9-40.0	≥40.1	F	P	≤12.6	12.7-26.7	26.8	≥35.5	13-36
13	≤20	21-24	≥25	≤38.4	38.5-39.6	≥39.7	F	P	≤13.3	13.4-27.7	27.8	≥36.3	14-37
14	≤22	23-26	≥27	≤38.1	38.2-39.3	≥39.4	F	P	≤13.9	14.0-28.5	28.6	≥36.8	15-39
15	≤25	26-29	≥30	≤37.8	37.9-39.0	≥39.1	F	P	≤14.5	14.6-29.1	29.2	≥37.1	16-40
16	≤27	28-31	≥32	≤37.6	37.7-38.8	≥38.9	F	P	≤15.2	15.3-29.7	29.8	≥37.4	17-41
17	≤30	31-34	≥35	≤37.5	37.6-38.7	≥38.8	F	P	≤15.8	15.9-30.4	30.5	≥37.9	18-42

Age (yr.)	Body mass index[c]				Flexed-arm hang (sec.)		Push-up (# completed)		Pull-up (# completed)		Modified pull-up (# completed)		Curl-up (# completed)	
	Very lean	HFZ	NI	NI (health risk)	NI	HFZ[c]	NI	HFZ[c]	NI	HFZ[e]	NI	HFZ[c]	NI	HFZ[c]
10	≤14.2	14.3-20.3	20.4	≥23.6	≤3	≥4	≤6	≥7	0	≥1	≤3	≥4	≤11	≥12
11	≤14.6	14.7-21.2	21.3	≥24.7	≤5	≥6	≤6	≥7	0	≥1	≤3	≥4	≤14	≥15
12	≤15.1	15.2-22.1	22.2	≥25.8	≤6	≥7	≤6	≥7	0	≥1	≤3	≥4	≤17	≥18
13	≤15.6	15.7-22.9	23.0	≥26.8	≤7	≥8	≤6	≥7	0	≥1	≤3	≥4	≤17	≥18
14	≤16.1	16.2-23.6	23.7	≥27.7	≤7	≥8	≤6	≥7	0	≥1	≤3	≥4	≤17	≥18
15	≤16.6	16.7-24.3	24.4	≥28.5	≤7	≥8	≤6	≥7	0	≥1	≤3	≥4	≤17	≥18
16	≤17.0	17.1-24.8	24.9	≥29.3	≤7	≥8	≤6	≥7	0	≥1	≤3	≥4	≤17	≥18
17	≤17.4	17.5-24.9	25.0	≥30.0	≤7	≥8	≤6	≥7	0	≥1	≤3	≥4	≤17	≥18

Age (yr.)	Trunk lift (in.)		Shoulder stretch (pass/fail)		Sit-and-reach (in.)	
	NI	HFZ[c]	NI	HFZ[c]	NI	HFZ[c]
10	≤8	9-12	F	P	≤8	9
11	≤8	9-12	F	P	≤9	10
12	≤8	9-12	F	P	≤9	10
13	≤8	9-12	F	P	≤9	10
14	≤8	9-12	F	P	≤9	10
15	≤8	9-12	F	P	≤11	12
16	≤8	9-12	F	P	≤11	12
17	≤8	9-12	F	P	≤11	12

a. NI and AFZ lap counts from Winnick and Short, 2014, developed with an equation provided by The Cooper Institute (2013). AFZ lap range represents a 3 percent reduction from V̇O₂max standard for the general population. Where appropriate, youngsters with visual impairment should pursue standards for the HFZ.

b. Reprinted, by permission, from The Cooper Institute, 2014, *Goal setting chart for aerobic capacity and PACER test*

c. Reprinted, by permission, from The Cooper Institute, 2013, *Fitnessgram/Activitygram test administration manual*, updated 4th ed. (Champaign, IL: Human Kinetics), 62.

d. Based on data from Project Target (1998).

e. Based on data from The Cooper Institute (1999).

f. The Cooper Institute, 2013, *Fitnessgram/Activitygram test administration manual*, updated 4th ed. (Champaign, IL: Human Kinetics), 66, 102.

Fitness Zone Table 7 Boys With Spinal Cord Injury

Age (yr.)	TAMT (pass/fail)		Percent body fat[b]				Triceps and calf skinfold[b,c] (mm)	Reverse curl (# completed)		Seated push-up (# completed)		Bench press (# completed)		Dumbbell press (# completed)	
	NI	HFZ[a]	Very lean	HFZ	NI	NI (health risk)	HFZ	NI	AFZ[a]	NI	AFZ[a]	NI	HFZ[a]	NI	HFZ[a]
10	F	P	≤8.8	8.9–22.4	22.5	≥33.2	11–29	0	≥1	≤4	≥5–20				
11	F	P	≤8.7	8.8–23.6	23.7	≥35.4	11–31	0	≥1	≤4	≥5–20				
12	F	P	≤8.3	8.4–23.6	23.7	≥35.9	10–31	0	≥1	≤4	≥5–20				
13	F	P	≤7.7	7.8–22.8	22.9	≥35.0	9–30	0	≥1	≤4	≥5–20	≤19	20–50	≤13	14–50
14	F	P	≤7.0	7.1–21.3	21.4	≥33.2	8–28	0	≥1	≤4	≥5–20	≤32	33–50	≤18	19–50
15	F	P	≤6.5	6.6–20.1	20.2	≥31.5	8–26	0	≥1	≤4	≥5–20	≤39	40–50	≤20	21–50
16	F	P	≤6.4	6.5–20.1	20.2	≥31.6	8–26	0	≥1	≤4	≥5–20	≤46	47–50	≤23	24–50
17	F	P	≤6.6	6.7–20.9	21.0	≥33.0	8–27	0	≥1	≤4	≥5–20	≤49	50	≤26	27–50

Age (yr.)	Grip strength (kg)		Modified Apley (score)		Modified Thomas (score)		Target stretch (score)	
	NI	HFZ[a]	NI	HFZ[a]	NI	HFZ[a]	NI	HFZ[a]
10	≤17	≥18	≤2	3	≤2	3	≤1	2
11	≤20	≥21	≤2	3	≤2	3	≤1	2
12	≤24	≥25	≤2	3	≤2	3	≤1	2
13	≤28	≥29	≤2	3	≤2	3	≤1	2
14	≤32	≥33	≤2	3	≤2	3	≤1	2
15	≤36	≥37	≤2	3	≤2	3	≤1	2
16	≤42	≥43	≤2	3	≤2	3	≤1	2
17	≤48	≥49	≤2	3	≤2	3	≤1	2

a. Based on data from Project Target (1998).

b. Reprinted, by permission, from The Cooper Institute, 2013, *Fitnessgram/Activitygram test administration manual*, updated 4th ed. (Champaign, IL: Human Kinetics), 61.

c. The Cooper Institute, 2013, *Fitnessgram/Activitygram test administration manual*, updated 4th ed. (Champaign, IL: Human Kinetics), 65, 101.

Fitness Zone Table 8 — Girls With Spinal Cord Injury

Age (yr.)	TAMT (pass/fail)		Percent body fat[b]				Triceps and calf skinfold[b,c] (mm)	Reverse curl (# completed)		Seated push-up (# completed)		Bench press (# completed)		Dumbbell press (# completed)	
	NI	HFZ[a]	Very lean	HFZ	NI	NI (health risk)	HFZ	NI	AFZ[a]	NI	AFZ[a]	NI	HFZ[a]	NI	HFZ[a]
10	F	P	≤11.5	11.6–24.3	24.4	≥33.0	11–32	0	≥1	≤4	≥5–20				
11	F	P	≤12.1	12.2–25.7	25.8	≥34.5	12–34	0	≥1	≤4	≥5–20				
12	F	P	≤12.6	12.7–26.7	26.8	≥35.5	13–36	0	≥1	≤4	≥5–20				
13	F	P	≤13.3	13.4–27.7	27.8	≥36.3	14–37	0	≥1	≤4	≥5–20	≤9	10–50	≤4	5–50
14	F	P	≤13.9	14.0–28.5	28.6	≥36.8	15–39	0	≥1	≤4	≥5–20	≤12	13–50	≤6	7–50
15	F	P	≤14.5	14.6–29.1	29.2	≥37.1	16–40	0	≥1	≤4	≥5–20	≤13	14–50	≤9	10–50
16	F	P	≤15.2	15.3–29.7	29.8	≥37.4	17–41	0	≥1	≤4	≥5–20	≤13	14–50	≤10	11–50
17	F	P	≤15.8	15.9–30.4	30.5	≥37.9	18–42	0	≥1	≤4	≥5–20	≤14	15–50	≤10	11–50

Age (yr.)	Grip strength (kg)		Modified Apley (score)		Modified Thomas (score)		Target stretch (score)	
	NI	HFZ[a]	NI	HFZ[a]	NI	HFZ[a]	NI	HFZ[a]
10	≤16	≥17	≤2	3	≤2	3	≤1	2
11	≤18	≥19	≤2	3	≤2	3	≤1	2
12	≤21	≥22	≤2	3	≤2	3	≤1	2
13	≤23	≥24	≤2	3	≤2	3	≤1	2
14	≤25	≥26	≤2	3	≤2	3	≤1	2
15	≤28	≥29	≤2	3	≤2	3	≤1	2
16	≤28	≥29	≤2	3	≤2	3	≤1	2
17	≤28	≥29	≤2	3	≤2	3	≤1	2

a. Based on data from Project Target (1998).

b. Reprinted, by permission, from The Cooper Institute, 2013, *Fitnessgram/Activitygram test administration manual*, updated 4th ed. (Champaign, IL: Human Kinetics), 62.

c. The Cooper Institute, 2013, *Fitnessgram/Activitygram test administration manual*, updated 4th ed. (Champaign, IL: Human Kinetics), 66, 102.

Fitness Zone Table 9   Boys With Cerebral Palsy

Age (yr.)	TAMT (pass/fail)		Percent body fat[b]				Triceps and calf skinfold[b,e] (mm)	Body mass index[b]				Seated push-up (# completed)	
	NI	HFZ[a]	Very lean	HFZ	NI	NI (health risk)	HFZ	Very lean	HFZ	NI	NI (health risk)	NI	AFZ[a]
10	F	P	≤8.8	8.9–22.4	22.5	≥33.2	11–29	≤14.4	14.5–19.7	19.8	≥22.7	≤4	≥5–20
11	F	P	≤8.7	8.8–23.6	23.7	≥35.4	11–31	≤14.8	14.9–20.5	20.6	≥23.7	≤4	≥5–20
12	F	P	≤8.3	8.4–23.6	23.7	≥35.9	10–31	≤15.2	15.3–21.3	21.4	≥24.7	≤4	≥5–20
13	F	P	≤7.7	7.8–22.8	22.9	≥35.0	9–30	≤15.7	15.8–22.2	22.3	≥25.6	≤4	≥5–20
14	F	P	≤7.0	7.1–21.3	21.4	≥33.2	8–28	≤16.3	16.4–23.0	23.1	≥26.5	≤4	≥5–20
15	F	P	≤6.5	6.6–20.1	20.2	≥31.5	8–26	≤16.8	16.9–23.7	23.8	≥27.2	≤4	≥5–20
16	F	P	≤6.4	6.5–20.1	20.2	≥31.6	8–26	≤17.4	17.5–24.5	24.6	≥27.9	≤4	≥5–20
17	F	P	≤6.6	6.7–20.9	21.0	≥33.0	8–27	≤18.0	18.1–24.9	25.0	≥28.6	≤4	≥5–20

Age (yr.)	40 m push/walk (pass/fail)		Wheelchair ramp test (feet)		Dumbbell press (# completed)		Grip strength (kg)		Modified Apley (score)		Modified Thomas (score)			Target stretch (score)		
	NI	AFZ[a]	NI	AFZ[a]	NI	HFZ[a]	NI	HFZ[a]	AFZ[c]	HFZ[a]	NI	AFZ[d]	HFZ[a]	NI	AFZ	HFZ[a]
10	F	P	≤7	≥8–15			≤17	≥18	2	3	≤1	2	3	0	1	2
11	F	P	≤7	≥8–15			≤20	≥21	2	3	≤1	2	3	0	1	2
12	F	P	≤7	≥8–15			≤24	≥25	2	3	≤1	2	3	0	1	2
13	F	P	≤7	≥8–15	≤13	14–50	≤28	≥29	2	3	≤1	2	3	0	1	2
14	F	P	≤7	≥8–15	≤18	19–50	≤32	≥33	2	3	≤1	2	3	0	1	2
15	F	P	≤7	≥8–15	≤20	21–50	≤36	≥37	2	3	≤1	2	3	0	1	2
16	F	P	≤7	≥8–15	≤23	24–50	≤42	≥43	2	3	≤1	2	3	0	1	2
17	F	P	≤7	≥8–15	≤26	27–50	≤48	≥49	2	3	≤1	2	3	0	1	2

a. Based on data from Project Target (1998).

b. Reprinted, by permission, from The Cooper Institute, 2013, *Fitnessgram/Activitygram test administration manual*, updated 4th ed. (Champaign, IL: Human Kinetics), 55.

c. AFZ is appropriate for classes C1 and C2L. When this test is recommended for other classes of cerebral palsy, use HFZ.

d. AFZ is appropriate for classes C5 and C7 (affected side). When this test is recommended for other classes of cerebral palsy, use HFZ.

e. The Cooper Institute, 2013, *Fitnessgram/Activitygram test administration manual*, updated 4th ed. (Champaign, IL: Human Kinetics), 65, 101.

Fitness Zone Table 10 Girls With Cerebral Palsy

Age (yr.)	TAMT (pass/fail)		Percent body fat[b]				Triceps and calf skinfold[b,e] (mm)	Body mass index[b]				Seated push-up (# completed)	
	NI	AFZ[a]	Very lean	HFZ	NI	NI (health risk)	HFZ	Very lean	HFZ	NI	NI (health risk)	NI	AFZ[a]
10	F	P	≤11.5	11.6–24.3	24.4	≥33.0	11–32	≤14.2	14.3–20.3	20.4	≥23.6	≤4	≥5–20
11	F	P	≤12.1	12.2–25.7	25.8	≥34.5	12–34	≤14.6	14.7–21.2	21.3	≥24.7	≤4	≥5–20
12	F	P	≤12.6	12.7–26.7	26.8	≥35.5	13–36	≤15.1	15.2–22.1	22.2	≥25.8	≤4	≥5–20
13	F	P	≤13.3	13.4–27.7	27.8	≥36.3	14–37	≤15.6	15.7–22.9	23.0	≥26.8	≤4	≥5–20
14	F	P	≤13.9	14.0–28.5	28.6	≥36.8	15–39	≤16.1	16.2–23.6	23.7	≥27.7	≤4	≥5–20
15	F	P	≤14.5	14.6–29.1	29.2	≥37.1	16–40	≤16.6	16.7–24.3	24.4	≥28.5	≤4	≥5–20
16	F	P	≤15.2	15.3–29.7	29.8	≥37.4	17–41	≤17.0	17.1–24.8	24.9	≥29.3	≤4	≥5–20
17	F	P	≤15.8	15.9–30.4	30.5	≥37.9	18–42	≤17.4	17.5–24.9	25.0	≥30.0	≤4	≥5–20

Age (yr.)	40 m push/walk (pass/fail)		Wheelchair ramp test (feet)		Dumbbell press (# completed)		Grip strength (kg)		Modified Apley (score)			Modified Thomas (score)			Target stretch (score)		
	NI	AFZ[a]	NI	AFZ[a]	NI	HFZ[a]	NI	HFZ[a]	NI	AFZ[c]	HFZ[a]	NI	AFZ[d]	HFZ[a]	NI	AFZ	HFZ[a]
10	F	P	≤7	≥8–15			≤16	≥17	≤1	2	3	≤1	2	3	0	1	2
11	F	P	≤7	≥8–15			≤18	≥19	≤1	2	3	≤1	2	3	0	1	2
12	F	P	≤7	≥8–15			≤21	≥22	≤1	2	3	≤1	2	3	0	1	2
13	F	P	≤7	≥8–15	≤4	5–50	≤23	≥24	≤1	2	3	≤1	2	3	0	1	2
14	F	P	≤7	≥8–15	≤6	7–50	≤25	≥26	≤1	2	3	≤1	2	3	0	1	2
15	F	P	≤7	≥8–15	≤9	10–50	≤28	≥29	≤1	2	3	≤1	2	3	0	1	2
16	F	P	≤7	≥8–15	≤10	11–50	≤28	≥29	≤1	2	3	≤1	2	3	0	1	2
17	F	P	≤7	≥8–15	≤10	11–50	≤28	≥29	≤1	2	3	≤1	2	3	0	1	2

a. Based on data from Project Target (1998).

b. Reprinted, by permission, from The Cooper Institute, 2013, Fitnessgram/Activitygram test administration manual, updated 4th ed. (Champaign, IL: Human Kinetics), 66.

c. AFZ is appropriate for classes C1 and C2L. When this test is recommended for other classes of cerebral palsy, use HFZ.

d. AFZ is appropriate for classes C5 and C7 (affected side). When this test is recommended for other classes of cerebral palsy, use HFZ.

e. The Cooper Institute, 2013, Fitnessgram/Activitygram test administration manual, updated 4th ed. (Champaign, IL: Human Kinetics), 66, 102.

Fitness Zone **Table 11** Boys With Congenital Anomaly or Amputation

Age (yr.)	PACER (20 m laps)		1-mile run[c,d] ($\dot{V}O_2MAX$)			TAMT (pass/fail)		Percent body fat[c]				Triceps and calf skinfold[c,f] (mm)		Seated push-up (# completed)	
	NI[a]	HFZ[b]	NI (health risk)	NI	HFZ	NI	HFZ[e]	Very lean	HFZ	NI	NI (health risk)	HFZ	NI	NI	AFZ[e]
10	≤16	≥17	≤37.3	37.4–40.1	≥40.2	F	P	≤8.8	8.9–22.4	22.5	≥33.2	11–29	≤4	≤4	≥5–20
11	≤19	≥20	≤37.3	37.4–40.1	≥40.2	F	P	≤8.7	8.8–23.6	23.7	≥35.4	11–31	≤4	≤4	≥5–20
12	≤22	≥23	≤37.6	37.7–40.2	≥40.3	F	P	≤8.3	8.4–23.6	23.7	≥35.9	10–31	≤4	≤4	≥5–20
13	≤28	≥29	≤38.6	38.7–41.0	≥41.1	F	P	≤7.7	7.8–22.8	22.9	≥35.0	9–30	≤4	≤4	≥5–20
14	≤35	≥36	≤39.6	39.7–42.4	≥42.5	F	P	≤7.0	7.1–21.3	21.4	≥33.2	8–28	≤4	≤4	≥5–20
15	≤41	≥42	≤40.6	40.7–43.5	≥43.6	F	P	≤6.5	6.6–20.1	20.2	≥31.5	8–26	≤4	≤4	≥5–20
16	≤46	≥47	≤41.0	41.1–44.0	≥44.1	F	P	≤6.4	6.5–20.1	20.2	≥31.6	8–26	≤4	≤4	≥5–20
17	≤49	≥50	≤41.2	41.3–44.1	≥44.2	F	P	≤6.6	6.7–20.9	21.0	≥33.0	8–27	≤4	≤4	≥5–20

Age (yr.)	Bench press (# completed)		Dumbbell press (# completed)		Grip strength (kg)		Curl-up (# completed)		Trunk lift (in.)		Modified Apley (score)		Shoulder stretch (pass/fail)		Sit-and-reach (in.)		Target stretch (score)	
	NI	HFZ[e]	NI	HFZ[e]	NI	HFZ[e]	NI	HFZ[c]	NI	HFZ[c]	NI	HFZ[e]	NI	HFZ[c]	NI	HFZ[c]	NI	HFZ[e]
10					≤17	≥18	≤11	≥12	≤8	9–12	2	3	F	P	≤7	8	≤1	2
11					≤20	≥21	≤14	≥15	≤8	9–12	2	3	F	P	≤7	8	≤1	2
12					≤24	≥25	≤17	≥18	≤8	9–12	2	3	F	P	≤7	8	≤1	2
13	≤19	20–50	≤13	14–50	≤28	≥29	≤20	≥21	≤8	9–12	2	3	F	P	≤7	8	≤1	2
14	≤32	33–50	≤18	19–50	≤32	≥33	≤23	≥24	≤8	9–12	2	3	F	P	≤7	8	≤1	2
15	≤39	40–50	≤20	21–50	≤36	≥37	≤23	≥24	≤8	9–12	2	3	F	P	≤7	8	≤1	2
16	≤46	47–50	≤23	24–50	≤42	≥43	≤23	≥24	≤8	9–12	2	3	F	P	≤7	8	≤1	2
17	≤49	50	≤26	27–50	≤48	≥49	≤23	≥24	≤8	9–12	2	3	F	P	≤7	8	≤1	2

a. Lap counts from Winnick and Short, 2014, developed with an equation provided by The Cooper Institute (2013).

b. Reprinted, by permission, from The Cooper Institute, 2014, *Goal setting chart for aerobic capacity and PACER test.*

c. Reprinted, by permission, from The Cooper Institute, 2013, *Fitnessgram/Activitygram test administration manual*, updated 4th ed. (Champaign, IL: Human Kinetics), 65.

d. Because the $\dot{V}O_2$max formula includes body mass index, $\dot{V}O_2$max will be overestimated if body mass index is not adjusted for the weight of a missing limb.

e. Based on data from Project Target (1998).

f. The Cooper Institute, 2013, *Fitnessgram/Activitygram test administration manual*, updated 4th ed. (Champaign, IL: Human Kinetics), 65, 101.

Fitness Zone Table 12 Girls With Congenital Anomaly or Amputation

Age (yr.)	PACER (20 m laps)		1-mile run (V̇O₂MAX)			TAMT (pass/fail)		Percent body fat				Triceps and calf skinfold (mm)	Seated push-up (# completed)	
	NI[a]	HFZ[b]	NI (health risk)	NI	HFZ	NI	HFZ[e]	Very lean	HFZ	NI	NI (health risk)	HFZ	NI	AFZ[e]
10	≤16	≥17	≤37.3	37.4–40.1	≥40.2	F	P	≤11.5	11.6–24.3	24.4	≥33.0	11–32	≤4	≥5–20
11	≤19	≥20	≤37.3	37.4–40.1	≥40.2	F	P	≤12.1	12.2–25.7	25.8	≥34.5	12–34	≤4	≥5–20
12	≤22	≥23	≤37.0	37.1–40.0	≥40.1	F	P	≤12.6	12.7–26.7	26.8	≥35.5	13–36	≤4	≥5–20
13	≤24	≥25	≤36.6	36.7–39.6	≥39.7	F	P	≤13.3	13.4–27.7	27.8	≥36.3	14–37	≤4	≥5–20
14	≤26	≥27	≤36.3	36.4–39.3	≥39.4	F	P	≤13.9	14.0–28.5	28.6	≥36.8	15–39	≤4	≥5–20
15	≤29	≥30	≤36.0	36.1–39.0	≥39.1	F	P	≤14.5	14.6–29.1	29.2	≥37.1	16–40	≤4	≥5–20
16	≤31	≥32	≤35.8	35.9–38.8	≥38.9	F	P	≤15.2	15.3–29.7	29.8	≥37.4	17–41	≤4	≥5–20
17	≤32	≥35	≤35.7	35.8–38.7	≥38.8	F	P	≤15.8	15.9–30.4	30.5	≥37.9	18–42	≤4	≥5–20

Age (yr.)	Bench press (# completed)		Dumbbell press (# completed)		Grip strength (kg)		Curl-up (# completed)		Trunk lift (in.)		Modified Apley (score)		Shoulder stretch (pass/fail)		Sit-and-reach (in.)		Target stretch (score)	
	NI	HFZ[e]	NI	HFZ[e]	NI	HFZ[e]	NI	HFZ[c]	NI	HFZ[c]	NI	HFZ[e]	NI	HFZ[c]	NI	HFZ[c]	NI	HFZ[e]
10					≤16	≥17	≤11	≥12	≤8	9–12	2	3	F	P	≤8	9	≤1	2
11					≤18	≥19	≤14	≥15	≤8	9–12	2	3	F	P	≤9	10	≤1	2
12					≤21	≥22	≤17	≥18	≤8	9–12	2	3	F	P	≤9	10	≤1	2
13	≤9	10–50	≤4	5–50	≤23	≥24	≤17	≥18	≤8	9–12	2	3	F	P	≤9	10	≤1	2
14	≤12	13–50	≤6	7–50	≤25	≥26	≤17	≥18	≤8	9–12	2	3	F	P	≤9	10	≤1	2
15	≤13	14–50	≤9	10–50	≤28	≥29	≤17	≥18	≤8	9–12	2	3	F	P	≤11	12	≤1	2
16	≤13	14–50	≤10	11–50	≤28	≥29	≤17	≥18	≤8	9–12	2	3	F	P	≤11	12	≤1	2
17	≤14	15–50	≤10	11–50	≤28	≥29	≤17	≥18	≤8	9–12	2	3	F	P	≤11	12	≤1	2

a. Lap counts from Winnick and Short, 2014, developed with an equation provided by The Cooper Institute (2013).

b. Reprinted, by permission, from The Cooper Institute, 2014, Goal setting chart for aerobic capacity and PACER test.

c. Reprinted, by permission, from The Cooper Institute, 2013, Fitnessgram/Activitygram test administration manual, updated 4th ed. (Champaign, IL: Human Kinetics), 66.

d. Because the V̇O₂max formula includes body mass index, V̇O₂max will be overestimated if body mass index is not adjusted for the weight of a missing limb.

e. Based on data from Project Target (1998).

f. The Cooper Institute, 2013, Fitnessgram/Activitygram test administration manual, updated 4th ed. (Champaign, IL: Human Kinetics), 66, 102.

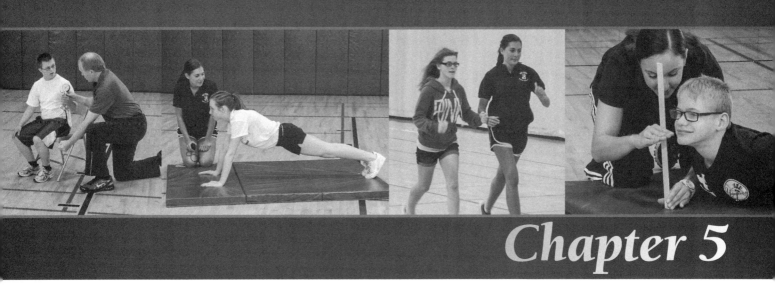

Chapter 5

Test Administration and Test Items

This chapter presents test items in the BPFT in detail, along with specific recommendations for administering most test items. Although the BPFT includes 27 test items, testers generally administer only 4 to 6 items to a particular individual. The following list provides general recommendations for administering the BPFT.

- Practice administering test items and be confident of your mastery in administering them before taking formal measurements.

- Develop forms for selecting test items and recording scores, or use materials developed as part of the Brockport Physical Fitness Test.

- Describe the test to participants and explain what it is intended to assess.

- Ensure that individuals being tested dress appropriately; exercise clothing and sneakers (where appropriate) are recommended.

- Plan and provide general and specific warm-ups, as appropriate. This is particularly important for test items involving flexibility or range of motion and strenuous effort.

- Provide cool-down activities after testing. This is especially important after aerobic-functioning test items.

- Provide a positive testing atmosphere. Encourage individuals being tested to try their best and continually provide positive reinforcement for effort.

- Compare participants' performances with criterion-referenced standards rather than with other individuals' performances.

- Administer no more than half of the items on a particular day. If fatigue appears to be influencing performance, provide longer rest intervals between test items.

- Administer aerobic-functioning tests last.

- Administer running items on a surface that is flat and hard yet resilient.

- Give participants who are blind the opportunity to become clearly oriented to a test

---

The Brockport Physical Fitness Test (BPFT) for youngsters with disability was designed to correspond as closely as possible to health-related, criterion-referenced tests for youngsters without disability. The BPFT corresponds most closely to Fitnessgram (Cooper Institute, 2013). To enhance consistency, the procedures for the following test items, which are also included in Fitnessgram, were adapted, by permission, from The Cooper Institute, 2013, *Fitnessgram/Activitygram test administration manual*, updated 4th ed. (Champaign, IL: Human Kinetics): PACER, one-mile run/walk, percent body fat, skinfolds, body mass index, curl-up, flexed-arm hang, pull-up, modified pull-up, push-up, shoulder stretch, trunk lift, back-saver sit-and-reach, and aerobic-capacity test items. The procedures for other test items were developed by Project Target and the authors of this book.

station or testing area. This is particularly important for tests that involve running.

- Provide careful demonstrations for participants with hearing impairment. Give instructions in writing or manually (e.g., signing, finger spelling). Use hand signals to start and stop activities.

- Administer the following test items individually to one participant at a time: target aerobic movement test (TAMT), percent body fat, skinfolds, extended-arm hang, flexed-arm hang, modified pull-up, pull-up, dominant grip strength, bench press, curl-up, modified curl-up, 40-meter push/walk, reverse curl, seated push-up, trunk lift, wheelchair ramp test, and most flexibility or range-of-motion test items (except shoulder stretch).

- The PACER, one-mile run/walk, and shoulder stretch may be administered to small groups of subjects at once. However, it may be necessary or most appropriate to provide partners for assistance.

- The following items can be administered to groups of two or three: dumbbell press, isometric push-up, and push-up. For the dumbbell press, provide spotters.

Safety Guidelines and Precautions

Test items used in connection with the BPFT (including nontraditional ones) are typical of those used elsewhere in physical education or physical fitness programs. Some have appeared on disability-specific tests of physical fitness or tests classifying athletes with disability or are associated with activities of daily living. Although the BPFT is considered safe, one must recognize that accidents are possible. Use the following guidelines and precautions when administering test items. Also adhere to guidelines for specific test items presented later in this chapter and to other recommended professional practices.

- Personnel who administer the test should be qualified and knowledgeable about physical fitness testing and disability.

- Maximize the safety of all youngsters. Professionals using this test should follow the policies of their school or agency regarding medical information, medical records, and medical clearance for activity. Any others should administer this test only following approval by a physician who is aware of the health status of the individual taking the test. Consider information from manufacturers of any test equipment used in conjunction with the BPFT.

- Avoid administering tests under conditions of unusually high or low temperature or humidity or when windy. Youngsters with spinal cord injury may be especially prone to problems with thermoregulation, including overheating.

- Be sure that individuals being tested understand test instructions. Provide opportunities for students to practice test items.

- Terminate the test item if the individual being tested experiences dizziness, pain, or disorientation.

- Avoid comparing individuals' performances with each other.

- Spot youngsters where necessary and appropriate.

- Incorporate warm-up and cool-down periods as appropriate for test items.

- Before testing, have youngsters with spinal cord injury above T6 empty their bowels and bladder and check them for tight clothing, straps, or pressure sores that might contribute to skin irritation. Individuals with spinal injury above T6 are subject to autonomic dysreflexia, a condition that can dangerously elevate the heart rate and blood pressure as a result of bowel or bladder distension or skin irritation.

- Be aware that some heart rate monitors may use latex in the strap, which can cause allergic reaction; therefore, wearing the strap may be contraindicated in certain instances.

Age Considerations

For purposes of the BPFT, the age of the individual being tested is determined on the date when the first test item is administered. Ages are not rounded to the nearest year. Thus, for example, an individual who is 10 years and 11 months old should be identified as being 10 years old.

Index of Test Items

Test items that have video clips in the accompanying web resource will be noted by the video icon placed next to the test title within the chapter. Use the pass code Brockport58743AR7 to access the web resource at www.HumanKinetics.com/BrockportPhysicalFitnessTestManual.

40-meter push/walk, page 82

Back-saver sit-and-reach, page 89

Bench press, page 69

Bioelectrical impedance analysis, page 68

Body mass index, page 67

Curl-up, page 70

Dominant grip strength, page 76

Dumbbell press, page 73

Extended-arm hang, page 74

Flexed-arm hang, page 75

Isometric push-up, page 77

Modified Apley test, page 88

Modified curl-up, page 72

Modified pull-up, page 79

Modified Thomas test, page 92

One-mile run/walk, page 63

PACER (20-meter and 15-meter), page 58

Pull-up, page 78

Push-up, page 80

Reverse curl, page 84

Seated push-up, page 85

Shoulder stretch, page 91

Skinfolds, page 65

Target aerobic movement test (TAMT), page 59

Target stretch test (TST), page 94

 Elbow extension, page 94

 Forearm pronation, page 95

 Forearm supination, page 95

 Knee extension, page 95

 Shoulder abduction, page 94

 Shoulder extension, page 94

 Shoulder external rotation, page 94

 Wrist extension, page 94

Trunk lift, page 86

Wheelchair ramp test, page 87

AEROBIC FUNCTIONING

PACER (20-Meter and 15-Meter)

In the PACER, participants run as long as possible back and forth across a distance of either 15 meters (16 yards, 15 inches) or 20 meters (21 yards, 32 inches) at a specified pace, which gets faster each minute. Designed to measure aerobic capacity, the test is conducted on a flat, nonslip surface. Participants run across the designated area to a line by the time a beep sounds from a recording. At the sound of the beep, they turn around and run back to the other end. If a participant reaches the line before the beep, he or she must wait for the next beep before running in the other direction. Participants continue in this manner until they can no longer reach the line before the beep sounds. Participants who do not reach the line before the beep sounds should be given two more beeps to regain the pace before being withdrawn. In attempting to catch up, the entire 15-meter or 20-meter lap must be completed. Upon completing the test, participants should walk from the testing area to a designated cool-down area, being careful not to interfere with others still running, and continue to walk and stretch in the cool-down area.

Equipment

Required equipment includes the PACER audio recording, an audio player with adequate volume, measuring tape, marker cones, a pencil, and score sheets. Participants should wear nonslip shoes. Plan for each participant to have a running space that is 40 to 60 inches (about 100 to 150 centimeters) wide. The PACER recording may include music or only the beeps.

Scoring and Trials

One test trial is given. The individual's score is the number of completed laps. When 15-meter lap scores are used, they must be converted to 20-meter-lap equivalents (see appendix D). A run of at least 10 laps (in the 20-meter version) is required in order to calculate aerobic capacity.

Test Modifications

Runners who are blind may run with assistance from a partner, with guide wire or rope assistance (see figure 5.1, a and b), trailing along a wall, or using other tactual assistance. Runners with an assisting partner can use a short tether rope or grasp the partner's elbow. In choosing a method of guidance, be sure that it does not inhibit running performance. For validity, give blind runners the opportunity to perform optimally. The runner should practice using the selected assistance until he or she is comfortable with it.

Be sure that youngsters with intellectual disability understand how to perform the test; take whatever time is necessary to ensure that participants learn the test. Because motivation is critical, at least one person should provide continual positive reinforcement to runners as they perform the test. Youngsters with intellectual disability often need to run with a tester or aide; however, assistants must not pull or push runners or give them any other physical advantage.

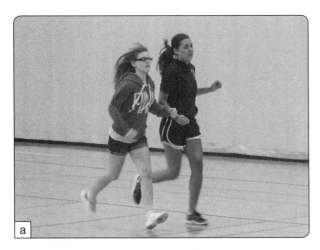
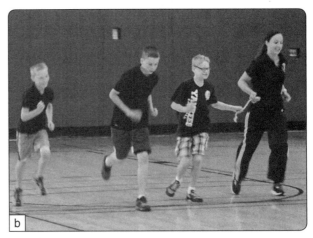

Figure 5.1 PACER test: (a) touching a sighted guide and (b) with guide-rope assistance.

AEROBIC FUNCTIONING

The PACER is preferred over the one-mile run particularly for youngsters with intellectual disability for shortest and slowest performances and when BMI is not to be incorporated in the calculation of $\dot{V}O_2max$. As participants exhibit increased mastery, the test may be modified so that they run laps in one direction only around a track or running surface to enhance preparation for long-distance running.

Suggestions for Test Administration

- Mark the PACER distance with marker cones and tape or chalk lines.

- Before test day, allow participants at least two practice sessions. Also allow participants to listen to several minutes of the audio recording before they perform the test so that they know what to expect.

- The test recording contains 21 levels (21 minutes). The 20-meter recording allows 9 seconds to run the distance during the first minute, and the pace increases by approximately half a second each following minute. The 15-meter recording allows 6.75 seconds to run the distance during the first minute, with lap time decreases of about half a second at each successive level.

- Single beeps indicate the end of a lap. Triple beeps at the end of each minute indicate an increase in speed. Participants should be alerted that the speed will increase. Caution participants not to begin too fast; the beginning speed is very slow.

- If a participant cannot reach the line before the beep sounds, he or she should be given two beeps to attempt to regain the pace before being withdrawn. If the participant regains the pace, continue to count laps. Give credit for a lap only if the entire PACER distance is completed.

- Volunteers can assist in recording scores.

- If participants are unable to hear beeps from the audio player, a whistle corresponding to the beeps can be used.

Target Aerobic Movement Test

The target aerobic movement test (TAMT) is a modification of the aerobic movement test developed by Pat Good at the Howe School in Dearborn, Michigan. It measures the aerobic behavior of youngsters and their ability to exercise at or above a recommended target heart rate (THR) for 15 minutes. The test is recommended for youngsters with certain disabilities and with the PACER serves as an optional test for students who are unable to perform the one-mile run/walk in 13 minutes or less. Exercises that can be used in the test include, for example, running, dancing, swimming, and arm ergometry. The test's basic level (level 1) estimates the ability to sustain a moderate intensity of physical activity (i.e., 70 percent of maximal predicted heart rate) without exceeding 85 percent of maximal predicted heart rate. Participants can engage in virtually any physical activity as long as it involves sufficient intensity to reach a minimal target heart rate and to sustain the heart rate in a target heart rate zone (THRZ). In preparation for the test, testers are encouraged to work with individuals to help them identify an appropriate physical activity.

For most participants—those who engage in whole-body forms of exercise (figure 5.2a)—the THRZ is defined as 70 percent to 85 percent of a maximal predicted heart rate (operationally, 140 to 180 beats per minute). Two exceptions exist. The first applies to participants with spinal cord injury resulting in low-level quadriplegia (LLQ, any spinal lesion between C6 and C8 inclusive). For these youngsters, THRZ may be defined in one of two ways. If an individual has a resting (sitting) heart rate of less than 65 beats per minute, the THRZ is defined as 85 to 100 beats per minute. If an individual's resting heart rate is 65 beats per minute or more, the THRZ is defined as a range of 20 to 30 beats above the resting value. For example, if an individual has a resting heart rate of 75 beats per minute, the THRZ will be 95 to 105 beats per minute. The second exception applies to those who engage in strictly arm exercise (figure 5.2b). For those who use arm-only exercise, the THRZ is 130 to 170 beats per minute.

The tester checks the participant's heart rate at least once every 60 seconds. If a participant is within his or her THRZ and no more than 10 beats above THR, the tester reinforces the behavior and

AEROBIC FUNCTIONING

encourages the participant to continue at the present intensity of exercise (e.g., "Nice job! Just keep doing what you've been doing at the same speed"). If a participant is below his or her THRZ, the tester encourages the participant to increase the exercise intensity (e.g., "Okay, your heart rate is a little low right now, so try to exercise a little harder or a little faster"). Should a participant fall below the THRZ, he or she has 1 minute to regain the minimal value. If the participant does so, the test continues; if not, the test is terminated. If the participant is above the THRZ the tester should acknowledge the participant's effort but also encourage the participant to decrease exercise intensity (e.g., "Wow, you're really working hard—in fact, a little too hard! Try to exercise a little lighter or a little slower"). If a participant works above the THRZ but completes the 15-minute test, his or her results can be considered as meeting the criterion. If a participant is beyond the THRZ for 2 or more consecutive minutes and fails to reach the 15-minute criterion, he or she should be retested at a later time and encouraged to work at a lower intensity for the purposes of the test.

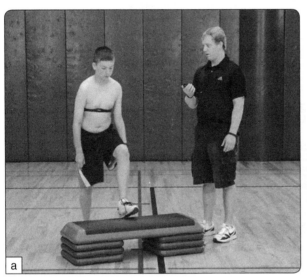 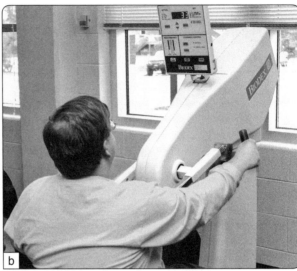

© BOLD STOCK / age fotostock

Figure 5.2 The target aerobic movement test: *(a)* whole-body form and *(b)* arm ergometry.

Equipment

This test item requires an exercise area large enough for adequate aerobic movement. It is also recommended that testers use an electronic heart rate monitor. If a monitor is not available, testers can choose an optional modified procedure using a stopwatch (or wristwatch that displays seconds). Music with a fast tempo is also recommended to provide motivation during the test and to encourage rhythmic, steady-state exercise.

Scoring and Trials

One test trial is given. This is a pass/fail test item; participants who can stay within or above the THRZ for 15 minutes pass the test. The 15-minute count begins when the participant enters the THRZ. For those unable to pass the test, it is recommended, for training purposes, that testers note how long the participant was able to exercise in the THRZ.

Test Modifications

If a heart rate monitor is unavailable, the test may be administered using the following procedures. The pulse rate at the wrist (i.e., radial pulse) is counted manually for 10-second intervals at a number of predetermined checkpoints. (The participant's exercise must be briefly interrupted for each pulse rate check.) Specifically, the pulse rate is checked at the end of a 3-minute warm-up period and at the end of each of the following exercise intervals after warm-up: 2 minutes, 4 minutes, 6 minutes, 9 minutes, 12 minutes, and 15 minutes. If the participant is below the minimum THRZ value at any checkpoint, he or she should be encouraged to increase the intensity of exercise and continue the test. If an individual is below the THRZ for two consecutive checkpoints, the test is terminated. Youngsters should be encouraged to maintain a steady exercise pace rather than fluctuate the exercise intensity. Minimal 10-second THRZ values and maximal THRZ values appear in table 5.1. It is recommended that the test be terminated if youngsters attain the maximal values during a warm-up or test period.

Table 5.1 Minimal and Maximal 10-Second Heart Rate (HR) Values

	Minimal	Maximal
General	23	30
Quadriplegic (C6–C8)		
Resting HR < 65	14	17
Resting HR ≥ 65	(Resting HR + 20) / 6	(Resting HR + 30) / 6
Arm-only exercise (paraplegic)	22	28

Participants who are able to exercise within these 10-second pulse rate values for 15 minutes (following a 3-minute warm-up) pass the test. If an individual cannot pass the test, the tester should note the approximate length of time for which the individual was in the THRZ based on the checkpoints. If a participant is below or above the THRZ at one checkpoint but regains the THRZ at the next checkpoint, the individual is credited for both checkpoints, and the test continues. If a participant works above his or her THRZ but completes the 15-minute test, his or her results can be considered as meeting the criteria as long as they do not go below the THRZ requirements. If a participant is below the THRZ for two consecutive checkpoints, however, the test ends, the participant is not credited for either checkpoint, and his or her score reverts to the last checkpoint within the THRZ.

The TAMT can also be used to measure the ability to sustain more vigorous physical activity. However, it is not recommended that higher-level intensities be used for people with quadriplegia. Table 5.2 summarizes THR and THRZ information by levels.

Table 5.2 Minimum Target Heart Rates (THRs) and Target Heart Rate Zones (THRZs) for TAMT Levels

Prescribed level of intensity	Minimum predicted heart rate intensity	Minimum THR and THRZ for whole-body activity	Minimum THR and THRZ for arm-only activity
1. Moderate	70%	140 (minimum THR)	130 (minimum THR)
		140–180 (THRZ)	130–170 (THRZ)
2. Low-level vigorous	75%	150 (minimum THR)	140 (minimum THR)
		150–180 (THRZ)	140–170 (THRZ)
3. Vigorous	80%	160 (minimum THR)	150 (minimum THR)
		160–180 (THRZ)	150–170 (THRZ)

Suggestions for Test Administration

- Provide a cool-down area and activities of decreasing intensity for participants at the conclusion of the test.
- In many cases, it will be necessary to lead up to the test by discussing the procedures with participants and providing training sessions of shorter duration than required by the test. One method is to start with a 5-minute training session and periodically increase the duration by 3-minute intervals until participants are ready for the full exercise period.
- Individuals with spinal injury above T6 are subject to autonomic dysreflexia, a condition that can elevate the heart rate and blood pressure as a result of bowel or bladder distension or skin irritation. As a precaution, therefore, it is recommended that youngsters with spinal cord injury above T6

empty their bowels and bladder before testing and be checked for tight clothing, straps, or pressure sores that might contribute to skin irritation.

- Some participants require braces (e.g., thoracolumbosacral orthoses or TLSO braces) during testing. Medical personnel need to be consulted to determine whether participation in the specific physical activity is permitted and whether the brace needs to be worn. If a brace is worn, care must be taken to develop an acceptable method for securing a heart rate monitor. For example, in certain instances it may be possible to loosen the back brace, place the transmitter under the brace, and then tighten the brace to keep the transmitter in place. If it is not possible to use a transmitter, the test modification of manual pulse rate counting may be required.

One-Mile Run/Walk

In this test, participants run or walk one mile (1,760 yards or 1,609 meters) in the shortest time possible. The test is used to measure aerobic capacity. Participants should be instructed to run or walk one mile at the fastest pace possible. The one-mile run/walk can be conducted on a track or any other flat, measured area—for example, a rectangle measuring 35 by 75 yards (32 by 68.6 meters), for which eight laps total one mile. Thus fields, playground areas, other grassy areas, and indoor courts can all be measured and marked to serve as an appropriate testing area.

Equipment

Required equipment includes a stopwatch, scorecards, pencils, and a clipboard.

Scoring and Trials

The one-mile run/walk is scored in minutes and seconds. One test trial is given. Note: In order to calculate aerobic capacity using the one-mile run/walk, height and weight for each student must be collected in addition to performance time. Aerobic capacity is not calculated on the basis of the one-mile run/walk for times over 13 minutes. When a participant's time is greater than 13 minutes, the tester should record and save the time as a measure of aerobic functioning and a baseline for comparison in future administrations of the test. Alternatively, testers may choose to give the PACER or TAMT to youngsters who are unable to run or walk a mile in less than 13 minutes.

Test Modifications

Runners who are blind may run with assistance from a partner. Assistance can involve using a short tether rope, touching or grasping the elbow of a sighted partner, or running alongside a sighted partner who gives verbal direction and encouragement (see figure 5.3). Once the method of ambulation is determined, ensure that it does not unduly inhibit running performance. For purposes of validity, a runner who is blind must be given the opportunity to perform optimally. The runner should practice using the selected method of assistance until he or she is comfortable with it.

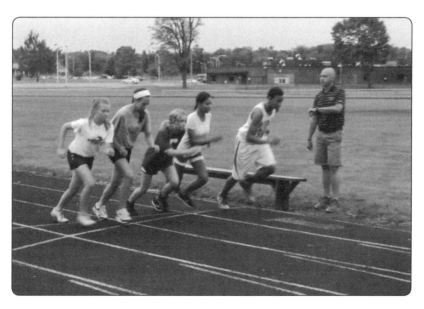

Figure 5.3 Running or walking the one-mile test.

Suggestions for Test Administration

- Before the day of testing, provide practice as necessary for the required distance.
- Participants should warm up properly before walking or running vigorously.
- Warm-up should include stretching exercises.
- It is recommended that youngsters not be tested in environments where temperature plus humidity is excessive.
- After test completion, give participants the opportunity to cool down by walking for several minutes.

Skinfolds

Skinfold tests determine the thickness of skinfolds at selected sites and can be used to estimate the body fat of youngsters. Skinfold measurements can be taken at three sites: triceps, subscapular, and calf. The triceps skinfold is taken over the triceps muscle at a location midway between the tip of the shoulder and the elbow (figure 5.4a). The subscapular skinfold is taken at a site approximately 1 inch (2.5 centimeters) below the tip of the scapula (inferior angle) and 1 inch toward the midline of the body (figure 5.4b). The calf skinfold is taken on the inside of the leg at about the level of maximal calf girth (figure 5.4c). The foot should be placed flat on an elevated surface with the knee flexed at a 90-degree angle. These measures should be taken on the participant's dominant or preferred side. Once the sites have been identified, the recommended testing procedure is as follows:

1. Grasp the skinfold firmly between the thumb and forefinger and pull slightly from the body, being careful to include only subcutaneous fat tissue, not muscle, in the fold. The triceps and calf skinfolds are vertical folds, while the subscapular skinfold is an oblique fold; see figure 5.4.

2. Place the tips of the caliper slightly (0.5 inch or 1.3 centimeters) above or below the fingers grasping the skinfold.

3. Slowly remove thumb pressure from the caliper, allowing it to exert full pressure on the fold.

4. Record the thickness of the fold to the nearest millimeter once the needle settles (1 to 2 seconds).

5. Open the caliper completely before removing it so as not to pinch the participant.

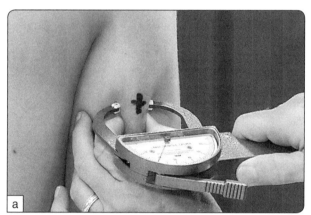

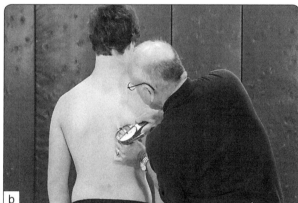

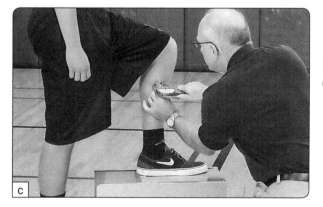

Figure 5.4 Skinfold measurements: *(a)* triceps, *(b)* subscapular, and *(c)* calf.

BODY COMPOSITION

BODY COMPOSITION

Equipment

A skinfold caliper of good quality should be used to obtain skinfold measurements (figure 5.5). The instrument should provide constant pressure on the skinfold of 10 grams per square millimeter.

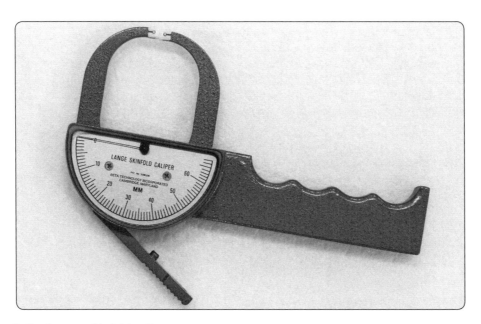

Figure 5.5 Lange skinfold caliper.
Photo courtesy of Matthew J. Yeoman.

Scoring and Trials

Three measurements should be taken at each selected skinfold site. The median (middle) score should be the criterion score. If a skinfold reading at the same site differs from other readings by 2 millimeters or more, an additional measurement should be taken, and the measurement that is substantially different should be ignored.

Test Modifications

Measurements should not be taken at sites with scar tissue, at sites where subdural or intramuscular injections have been received repeatedly, or on limbs that have muscular atrophy. In some instances, it may not be possible to attain skinfold measurements at a site.

Suggestions for Test Administration

- Testers should master administering the skinfold test before using it.
- Testers can help distinguish muscle and fat by having participants tense and relax the triceps muscle.
- The subscapular skinfold is an oblique fold, in line with the natural cleavage lines of the skin. Testers may be aided in finding the line by having subjects bend the elbow and place the arm on the back so that the back of the hand touches the spine while standing. The top of the fold should be medial to the bottom of the fold.
- It is recommended that females being tested wear a thin T-shirt or similar garment for measuring the subscapular skinfold. The shirt can be raised to allow access to the skinfold sites, or the measurement can be taken over the shirt. In such an instance, it would be necessary to subtract the fold of the T-shirt. For females wearing bras, the strap should be pushed upward only 2 to 3 inches (5 to 8 centimeters) to allow the measurement. If possible, female subjects should be measured by women.
- It is recommended that one measurement be taken at each site before taking second and third measurements at any site.

Body Mass Index

Whereas skinfolds estimate body fatness, body mass index reflects fat, muscle, and bone mass and indicates the appropriateness of an individual's weight for his or her height. Therefore, in order to compute BMI, height and weight must be determined.

Equipment

A scale is required, and a stadiometer is preferred. If a stadiometer is unavailable, a marked wall or tape measure can be used to determine height (or body length). Participants may lie on a mat to determine body height if they are unable to support their weight in a standing position.

Scoring and Trials

Only one measurement each is necessary for height and weight. Participants should wear lightweight clothing and remove shoes when possible. Initially, height can be rounded to the nearest half inch (whole centimeter) and weight to the nearest pound (half kilogram). BMI can be determined by using the chart presented in appendix A or by using the following equations:

$$BMI = \text{body weight (kilograms)} / \text{height}^2 \text{ (meters)}$$
$$BMI = \text{body weight (pounds)} \times 704.5 / \text{height}^2 \text{ (inches)}$$

To convert pounds to kilograms, divide by 2.2. To convert inches to meters, divide by 39.37. For example, consider a 170-pound person who is 5 feet 10 inches (70 inches) tall. The person's metric weight is 77.3 kilograms (170 pounds divided by 2.2), and his or her metric height is 1.8 meters (70 inches divided by 39.37). The person's BMI is calculated as 24 using either the metric or the English equation:

$$BMI = 77.3 \text{ (kilograms)} / 1.8^2 \text{ (meters)} = 77.3 / 3.2 = 24$$
$$BMI = 170 \text{ (pounds)} \times 704.5 / 70^2 \text{ (inches)} = 119{,}765 / 4{,}900 = 24$$

Test Modifications

The height of an individual who wears prosthetic devices or braces should be taken while he or she wears the items. Subjects who are unable to support their body weight in a standing position can lie on a mat while body length is measured with a tape measure. If an individual with cerebral palsy cannot stand erect because of exaggerated flexor tone in the hips or knees, the tester can use a tape to measure body segments (i.e., floor to knee, knee to hip, hip to head) and add the segments to determine body length for the purpose of calculating BMI.

The weight of an individual who wears a prosthetic device or brace is taken with the items removed or by subtracting the weight of the item. The weight of an individual who uses a wheelchair can be determined either by taking the individual out of the wheelchair or by weighing the individual in the wheelchair and then subtracting the weight of the wheelchair. Individuals with amputation or congenital anomaly can be weighed, but care must be taken when making comparisons with other people or calculating BMI. When estimating the weight of a person with a leg amputation, add 1/18 of body weight for a below-knee amputation, 1/9 of body weight for an above-knee amputation, and 1/6 of body weight for a hip amputation.

Suggestions for Test Administration

This test may be waived if determination of either height or weight poses a safety problem to the subject or the tester; if anomaly, amputation, or contracture prohibits valid measurement; or if BMI will not be used for assessment or program planning.

BODY COMPOSITION

Bioelectrical Impedance Analysis

Improvements in technology and cost have made it possible to provide portable bioelectrical impedance analysis (BIA) devices to accurately estimate body composition, specifically percent body fat. In this approach, body fat percentage is determined by measuring the body's resistance to electrical flow. A body with a higher percentage of muscle has greater total body water and lower resistance to electrical flow; on the other hand, a body with a higher percentage of fat has less body water and greater resistance to electrical flow. Depending on the particular BIA instrument used, the tester can determine height, weight, body mass index, and percentage of body fat relative to overall body weight.

The basic principle underlying BIA involves the resistance between two conductors attached to a person's body, and error can be caused by incorrect placement of the conductors. The test can also be affected by drinking and exercise, which affect hydration; for instance, an individual who consumes a large amount of water before the test may test out at a lowered body fat percentage.

Using BIA offers advantages, particularly when working with large numbers of school students. Results can be determined and recorded quickly—and much faster than is possible with skinfold measures. The procedure is also less invasive than taking skinfolds and thereby provides an excellent alternative to them. However, careful attention must be given to the methods of use described by BIA device manufacturers. Important before purchase is information regarding the psychometric qualities (reliability and validity) of the instrument. BIA is considered safe, but it should not be used without prior medical approval for persons with cardiac pacemakers, electrocardiographs, or other medical devices implanted in the body or used for life support.

Bench Press

This test item and its procedures were modified from Johnson and Lavay (1989). In it, participants perform as many bench presses as possible (to a maximum of 50 for males and 30 for females). The test is designed as a measure of upper-extremity (particularly elbow-extension) strength and endurance.

The participant lies supine on a bench with knees bent and feet on the floor or on rolled mats placed on either side of the bench. Individuals who are unable to assume this position should lie on the bench with knees flexed and lower extremities secured or supported. For safety, the tester acts as a spotter or assigns spotters (figure 5.6a). The participant grasps a 35-pound (15.9-kilogram) barbell with both hands directly above the shoulders and with elbows flexed; this is the ready position (figure 5.6b). Hands on the bar should be about shoulder-width apart with thumbs wrapped around the bar.

On command, the participant raises the barbell to a straight-arm position at a 90-degree angle to the body (figure 5.6c), then returns to the ready position. The participant repeats this action without rest until he or she can no longer raise the barbell or has successfully completed 50 repetitions for males or 30 repetitions for females. One repetition should be completed every 3 to 4 seconds at a steady pace. Spotters stand beside and adjacent to the rib cage, rather than behind the participant, so that the participant is encouraged to lift the barbell straight upward. Although a bilateral action with both arms is encouraged, the participant is credited with a successful repetition if the barbell touches the chest and both arms eventually end up in a straight-arm position without rest. The tester encourages the participant through praise and counting of repetitions.

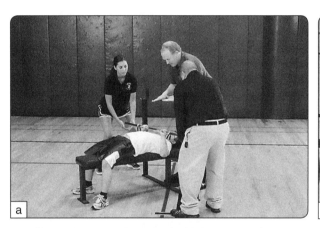

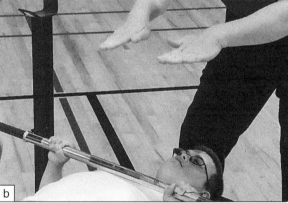

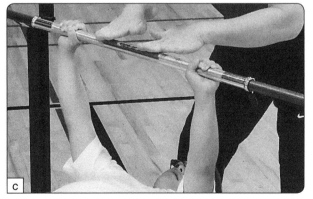

Figure 5.6 Bench press: *(a)* setting an upward target, *(b)* ready position, and *(c)* up position.

Equipment

Required equipment includes barbells and weights that together weigh 35 pounds (15.9 kilograms). A sturdy bench is recommended; the bench may be placed on a mat (optional).

Scoring and Trials

One correct bench press involves bringing the barbell from the chest to the straight-arm position. Record the number of correct bench press repetitions performed. Participants stop when they can no longer lift the weight completely or when they complete the required number of correct repetitions (50 for males, 30 for females).

Test Modifications

Be certain that participants with intellectual disability and mild limitations in physical fitness understand how to perform the test. Take whatever time is necessary for the participant to learn the test. Subjects should have the upper-body ability to perform the test. Provide those who have lower-body disability with safe and stable support while they assume the supine position on the bench. Participants can be held or secured as necessary and appropriate for stability.

Suggestions for Test Administration

- Conduct practice sessions with participants to help them understand the proper method for performing the bench press. Stress safety in a positive manner through demonstrations.
- Demonstrate and let participants experiment with the proper method of performing the bench press—first with a broomstick, then the bar only, then the bar and lighter weights, and finally the 35-pound (15.9-kilogram) barbell. At the same time, demonstrate and let participants experience the proper position for lying on the bench, proper hand position on the bar, proper leg and foot position, and correct arm movement. Setting an upward target enhances proper upward movement of the bar (figure 5.6c). Give positive reinforcement for properly executed positions and movements. Do not test a participant who does not understand how to complete a properly performed repetition of the bench press.

Curl-Up 🎥

In this test, participants complete as many curl-ups as possible, up to a maximum of 75, at a cadence of one curl every 3 seconds. The test is designed to measure abdominal strength and endurance. The participant starts by lying in a supine position on a mat. The knees are bent at an angle of approximately 140 degrees, with the feet flat on the floor and the legs slightly apart. The arms are held straight, parallel to the trunk, with the palms facing down toward the mat and the fingers outstretched. The participant is positioned so that the closest edge of a flat measuring strip that is 4.5 inches (about 11.5 centimeters) wide can be touched with the outstretched fingers (figure 5.7a).

From the starting position, the participant curls up slowly, sliding the fingers across and to the opposite side of the measuring strip (figure 5.7b). The participant then returns to the starting position. The important factor is that participants move the fingertips 4.5 inches (11.5 centimeters) as part of the curl-up. The tester should call the cadence (about one curl every 3 seconds). The participant continues without pausing until he or she either cannot maintain the pace or has completed 75 repetitions.

Equipment

The test uses a gym mat and a measuring strip that is 30 inches by 4.5 inches (76 centimeters by 11.5 centimeters). The measuring strip can be held or secured to a supporting surface. Although measuring strips made from cardboard or sanded plywood are recommended, other systems are acceptable for measuring the 4.5 inches. For example, tape markers can be placed on a mat to indicate start and finish points.

Scoring and Trials

One trial is administered. An individual's score is the number of curl-ups performed correctly. One curl-up is counted for every return to a supine position on the mat. Curl-ups should not be counted if

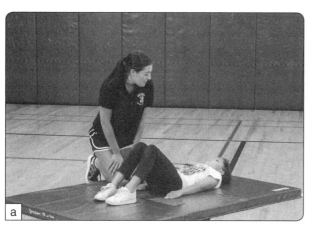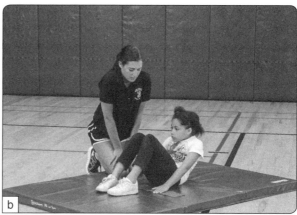

Figure 5.7 Curl-up: *(a)* starting position and *(b)* up position.

the feet completely leave the floor at any time during the movement or if the participant does not reach the required distance, does not return to the start position, or performs the curl-up in any other incorrect manner.

Test Modifications

It is acceptable to take whatever time is needed to ensure that youngsters know how to perform the test. Motivation is critical; therefore, continual positive reinforcement should be provided throughout testing.

Suggestions for Test Administration

- Encourage a slow curling of the upper spine during the curl-up.
- Encourage steady, controlled, and continuous movement.
- It may be necessary for an assistant to secure the measuring strip.
- Time can be saved by taping a measuring strip to a large mat and adjusting the participant's starting position to the measuring strip.
- A testing assistant can judge whether the participant's head touches the mat on each repetition with this judgment.

MUSCULOSKELETAL FUNCTIONING: MUSCULAR STRENGTH AND ENDURANCE

Modified Curl-Up

The modified curl-up uses the procedure recommended for the curl-up with the following exceptions:

- The hands are placed on the front of the thighs rather than on the mat alongside the body.
- As the participant curls up, the hands slide along the thighs until the fingertips contact the patellae (figure 5.8a). The hands should slide approximately 4 inches (10 centimeters) to the patellae or, if necessary, beyond.
- If necessary, testers can place their hands on the individual's kneecaps to provide a more tangible target for the individual's reach (figure 5.8b).

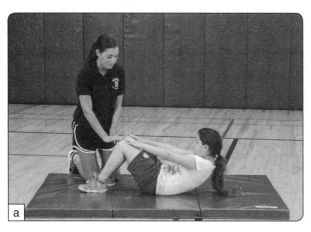 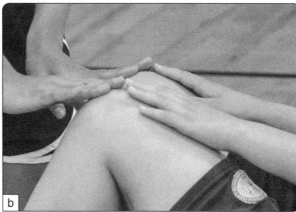

Figure 5.8 Modified curl-up: (a) hands sliding to the patellae; (b) setting a target.

Dumbbell Press 🎥

In this test, the participant lifts a 15-pound (6.8-kilogram) dumbbell as many times as possible, up to 50 repetitions, in a specific cadence. The test is designed to measure arm and shoulder strength and endurance. The participant is seated in a wheelchair or other sturdy chair (figure 5.9). For safety, the tester serves as a spotter or assigns spotters. The participant grasps the dumbbell with the dominant hand, with the elbow flexed so that the weight is close to and slightly in front of the dominant shoulder (figure 5.9a). Once the participant has control of the weight, he or she should extend the elbow and flex the shoulder so that the weight is lifted straight up and above the shoulder (figure 5.9b). When the elbow is completely extended, the participant returns the weight to the starting position. The exercise is continued at a steady pace (3 to 4 seconds per repetition) until the participant either completes 50 repetitions or is no longer able to lift the weight above the shoulder with complete elbow extension.

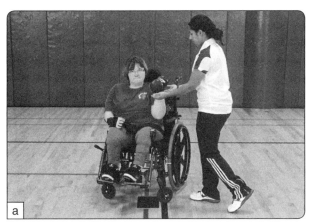
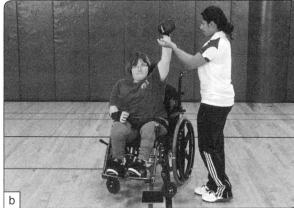

Figure 5.9 Dumbbell press: *(a)* starting position and *(b)* raised position.

Equipment

This test requires a 15-pound (6.8-kilogram) dumbbell, a stopwatch, and a wheelchair or other sturdy chair (preferably made of wood or metal).

Scoring and Trials

The participant receives one trial only. One successful lift is counted each time the dumbbell is raised above the shoulder with complete elbow extension. The scoring ends when the participant completes 50 repetitions, rests for more than 4 seconds between repetitions, or is unable to lift the weight with complete elbow extension.

Test Modifications

The test can be administered within the participant's range of motion. If complete elbow extension is not possible due to impairment, the tester should record a successful lift each time the participant lifts the weight with his or her maximal elbow range of motion. During the test, a steady pace should be emphasized. If a participant requires more than 4 seconds to complete a repetition because of a disability, this should be permitted as long as the participant is working to lift the weight.

Suggestions for Test Administration

- Before testing, be sure the participant understands how to execute the movement.
- Provide continual encouragement throughout the test.
- Match counting with a cadence. For example, say "one and down, two and down . . ." to prompt about one repetition every 3 to 4 seconds.

MUSCULOSKELETAL FUNCTIONING: MUSCULAR STRENGTH AND ENDURANCE

MUSCULOSKELETAL FUNCTIONING: MUSCULAR STRENGTH AND ENDURANCE

Extended-Arm Hang

In this test, the participant hangs from a bar or similar apparatus for as long as possible, up to 40 seconds. The test is designed to measure hand, arm, and shoulder strength and endurance. The participant begins by grasping the bar using an overhand, or pronated, grip (knuckles toward the face; see figure 5.10). The thumbs should be wrapped around the bar. The participant may jump to this position, be lifted to it, or move to it from a chair. The participant must assume a fully extended position with feet clear of the floor throughout the test. Elbows and knees must not be bent. The participant can be steadied so that he or she does not sway.

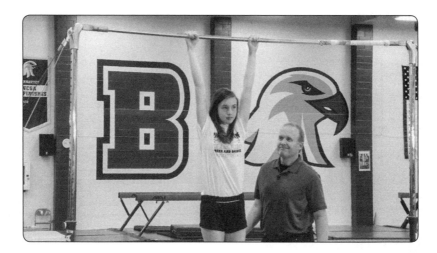

Figure 5.10 Extended-arm hang.

Equipment

This test item requires an adjustable bar about 1.5 inches (3.8 centimeters) in diameter at a height enabling performance without touching the support surface. The surface should be no more than 2 feet (0.6 meter) below the feet while the participant is in the hanging position. A gym mat should be placed under the bar. A stopwatch is required.

Scoring and Trials

One trial is permitted for each participant. The score is the elapsed time in seconds (to the nearest second) from the start of a free hang to the time that the fingers leave the bar.

Test Modifications

Individuals with disability must be provided with an opportunity to learn and experience the test item before scores are recorded for testing purposes.

Suggestions for Test Administration

- Be sure that the bar and the participant's hands are dry.
- Constant encouragement is extremely important throughout this test.
- For youngsters who are afraid of falling, keep them as close to the floor or ground as possible. Gently steady them, and assure them that they will be assisted if they lose their grip.

Flexed-Arm Hang

In this test, the participant maintains a flexed-arm position while hanging from a bar for as long as possible. The test is designed to measure hand, arm, and shoulder strength and endurance. The participant should grasp the bar with an overhand grip and be assisted to a position where the body is close to the bar and the chin is clearly over, but not touching, the bar (figure 5.11). The participant holds this position for as long as possible. The body must not swing, the knees must not be bent, and the legs must not kick during performance of the task. If a physical disability prohibits grasping, weight bearing, or reasonable execution, this item should not be administered.

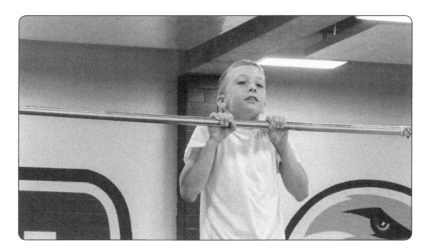

Figure 5.11   Flexed-arm hang.

Equipment

This test item requires a pull-up bar about 1.5 inches (3.8 centimeters) in diameter at a height exceeding the height of the participant, preferably no more than 3 feet (0.9 meter) and no less than 1.5 feet (0.45 meter) above the participant's standing height. A gym mat should be placed under the bar. A stopwatch is required.

Scoring and Trials

Each participant receives one trial. The tester records the length of time (to the nearest second) for which the participant maintains the flexed-arm position. Timing stops when the head tilts back or the chin contacts or drops below the bar.

Test Modifications

None.

Suggestions for Test Administration

- A spotter can place an arm across the participant's thighs to restrict unwanted movement.
- Be sure that the participant understands how to perform the test before taking a score. Provide sufficient time for the participant to learn the activity.

MUSCULOSKELETAL FUNCTIONING: MUSCULAR STRENGTH AND ENDURANCE

Dominant Grip Strength

In this test, participants squeeze a grip dynamometer with the stronger hand to generate as much force as possible. The test is designed to measure hand and arm strength. The participant should be seated on a straight-backed, armless chair with his or her feet flat on the floor. The tester must first adjust the handle of the dynamometer to fit the hand of the participant; when the dynamometer is squeezed, the second phalanx should rest on the adjustable handle. Once the dynamometer has been adjusted to the correct position, the participant should be instructed to squeeze the handle as hard as possible (figure 5.12). The hand grasping the dynamometer should be held away from the body and chair during the test.

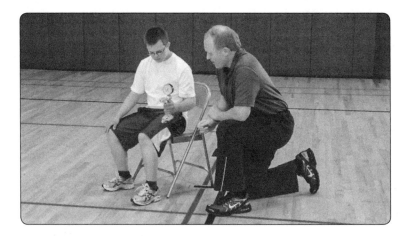

Figure 5.12   Dominant grip strength.

Equipment

Testers should use a good-quality grip dynamometer with an adjustable handle (figure 5.13). Data for this test presented in the tables found in chapter 4 were collected using a Jamar grip dynamometer.

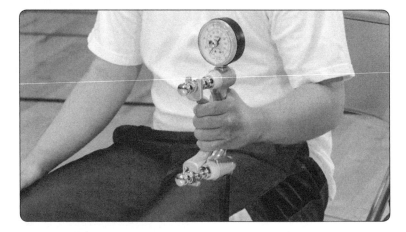

Figure 5.13   Grip dynamometer.

Scoring and Trials

Three trials are administered using the participant's preferred (stronger) hand. Allow at least 30 seconds between trials. After each trial, the needle should be reset to zero. The tester records each participant's score to the nearest kilogram. The middle score of the three trials serves as the criterion score.

Test Modifications

The dominant grip strength test item should not be administered to individuals without sufficient functional strength or to those unable to grasp or release because of an impairment. Participants can be seated in a wheelchair or on another support surface as long as the test can be administered appropriately.

Suggestions for Test Administration

- All participants must be motivated to enhance maximal effort.
- Do not test subjects until they have learned to perform the test properly.
- Individuals with intellectual disability must be given an opportunity to practice using the equipment and be taught the concept of squeezing with as much force as possible.

Isometric Push-Up

This test item and its procedures were modified from Johnson and Lavay (1989). The participant attempts to hold a raised push-up position for as long as 40 seconds. The test is designed primarily to measure upper-body strength and endurance. The participant assumes a front-leaning rest position with the hands directly below the shoulders, the arms extended, the whole body in a straight line, and the toes touching the floor or mat; this is the correct up position for a push-up (figure 5.14). The test is terminated when any movement—such as bending, sagging, or swaying—occurs at the elbows, shoulders, trunk, or knees. In other words, scoring is terminated when the correct up position for the push-up is no longer held.

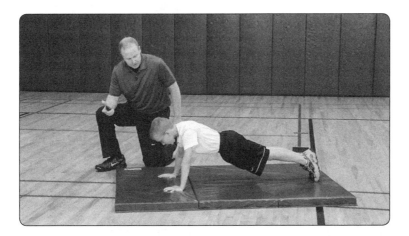

Figure 5.14 Isometric push-up.

**MUSCULOSKELETAL FUNCTIONING:
MUSCULAR STRENGTH AND ENDURANCE**

Equipment

This test requires a stopwatch and a flat, solid surface. A firm mat is recommended.

Scoring and Trials

One test trial is given. The tester records the length of time, to the nearest second, for which the participant holds the proper position.

Test Modifications

It is permissible to provide tactual assistance to help place and keep the body in the proper position during the test. However, no assistance should be given in holding the body upright.

Suggestions for Test Administration

- Do not test a participant who does not understand how to properly execute the isometric push-up.
- Take whatever time is necessary to ensure that participants learn the test.
- Since motivation is critical, provide continual positive reinforcement to each participant.
- Demonstrate and let participants experiment with the proper method of performing an isometric push-up, including the proper positions for hands, arms, head, trunk, legs, and feet. Give visual, verbal, and physical support prompts to help participants learn the correct position. Physical supports during testing are not permitted.

Pull-Up

In this test, participants complete as many pull-ups as they can. The test is designed to measure upper-body strength and endurance. The participant begins in the position of a straight-arm hang from a bar using an overhand (pronated) grip (figure 5.15a). The participant then pulls the body up toward the bar until the chin is above the bar (figure 5.15b). Once this position is reached, the body is lowered to the full-hang starting position. The body must not swing, the knees must not be bent, and the legs must not kick during performance of the task.

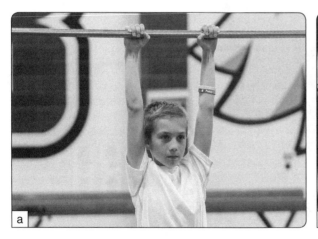
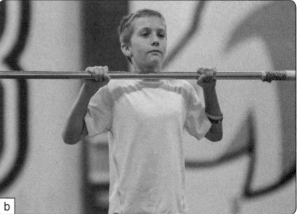

Figure 5.15 Pull-up: *(a)* down position and *(b)* up position.
Photos courtesy of Matthew J. Yeoman.

Equipment

This test uses a sturdy horizontal bar about 1.5 inches (3.8 centimeters) in diameter that permits the participant to hang with arms fully extended and feet not touching the floor. A gym mat should be placed under the bar.

Scoring and Trials

Each participant is permitted one trial, and the score attained is the number of pull-ups performed. There is no time limit for the test, but participants should be encouraged to complete the test quickly in order to reduce the effects of fatigue.

Test Modifications

Testing assistants may need to spot participants in order to reduce the possibility of falling or losing balance after falling from bar.

Suggestions for Test Administration

- Be sure that the participant understands how to perform the test before taking a score. Provide sufficient time for the participant to learn to perform the test item with confidence.
- Spotters may place an arm across the participant's thighs to restrict swinging of the body, kicking, or other unwanted movement during the task.

Modified Pull-Up

In this test, participants execute as many pull-ups as possible using a pull-up stand. The test is a measure of upper-body strength and endurance. It uses a modified pull-up apparatus (see appendix B and figure 5.16). The participant lies down under the crossbar so that the bar is directly over the shoulders. The participant's arms are extended up toward the bar, which should be set 1 to 2 inches (2.5 to 5 centimeters) above the participant's outstretched arms. An elastic band is placed on a peg 7 to 8 inches (18 to 20 centimeters) below the bar. This band marks the height to which the participant's chin must rise for completion of one repetition.

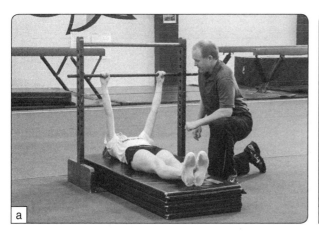 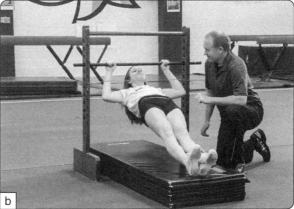

Figure 5.16 Modified pull-up: *(a)* starting position and *(b)* raised position.

MUSCULOSKELETAL FUNCTIONING: MUSCULAR STRENGTH AND ENDURANCE

To get into the starting position, the participant raises the body high enough to grasp the bar using an overhand (pronated) grip with thumbs around the bar. The pull-up begins in the down position with arms, legs, and body straight; buttocks off the floor; and only the heels touching the floor.

The pull-up action should raise the body to a height where the chin rises above the elastic band. Then the participant lowers to the starting position and repeats as many times as possible. Movement is performed using the arms only.

Equipment

A modified pull-up stand is preferred, but any adjustable bar arrangement can be used as long as the proper procedures are followed.

Scoring and Trials

The score is the number of correct pull-ups completed. There is no time limit, but the action should be continuous.

Test Modifications

Participants should be given sufficient practice to learn the test procedure.

Suggestions for Test Administration

- Give encouragement and positive feedback throughout the test.
- Stop the test if the participant experiences extreme discomfort.

Push-Up

In this test, participants complete as many push-ups as possible at a rate of 1 push-up every 3 seconds. The test is designed primarily to measure upper-body strength and endurance. To begin, the participant assumes a prone position on a mat with the hands placed under the shoulders, the fingers outstretched, the legs straight and slightly apart, and the weight on the tucked toes. The participant pushes to the up position until the arms are straight (figure 5.17a). Next, the participant lowers the body by bending the elbows to a 90-degree angle (figure 5.17b). The participant then returns to the straight-arm position. The cadence should be approximately 1 push-up every 3 seconds.

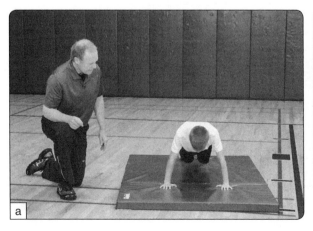 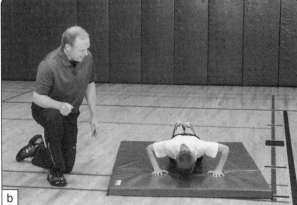

Figure 5.17   Push-up: *(a)* up position and *(b)* down position.

Equipment

Only a mat is required. However, in order to maintain good cadence, it is also recommended that testers use a watch with a second hand (by which cadence can be called out), a metronome, or an audio recording with the correct cadence.

Scoring and Trials

After learning the test, one trial is permitted. A participant's score is the number of correctly executed push-ups. The starting position for the push-up is the up position with the arms straight. One push-up is counted each time the participant bends the arms and returns to the straight-arm position. The test is terminated if the participant is unable to maintain correct cadence, stops to rest, or discontinues the activity. Push-ups done incorrectly should not be counted. Push-ups are incorrect if the knees touch the floor, the arms are not straight in the up position, the arms are not bent at 90 degrees on the downward movement, movement is jerky or not coordinated bilaterally, or the back is not kept reasonably straight.

Test Modifications

- Extra time should be provided for participants with intellectual disability to learn the test.
- Some latitude is recommended in performing to a cadence, that is, approximately 20 push-ups in 1 minute.
- Considerable time is required to teach the test to individuals with visual disability if they have not already learned how to perform a push-up. Provide tactual or kinesthetic cues to help participants know correct arm positions and recognize a straight back during the push-up.

Suggestions for Test Administration

- Be sure that all participants have time to learn to perform the test correctly.
- Encourage participants to breathe as they perform the activity, preferably exhaling while rising to the up position.
- To help participants learn the push-up, have them watch themselves in a mirror. This is especially important for learning to bend the elbows to 90 degrees and keeping the back straight in the up position.
- Have participants practice with a cadence.

MUSCULOSKELETAL FUNCTIONING: MUSCULAR STRENGTH AND ENDURANCE

40-Meter Push/Walk

In this test, participants walk or push their wheelchairs a distance of 40 meters (43 yards, 27 inches), after moving through a start zone of 5 meters (5 yards, 17 inches) at a speed that is comfortable for them (figure 5.18). This test item is designed to measure whether participants have the strength and endurance to traverse a distance of 40 meters without reaching a moderate level of exertion. This is not a dash or race, and testers should not emphasize high speed as a component of the test. Participants should be encouraged to travel at the speed they usually use for mobility in the community. To pass the test, participants must be able to cover the 40-meter distance in 60 seconds or less while keeping the heart rate below the criterion for moderate exercise intensity.

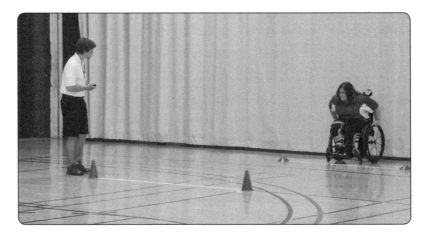

Figure 5.18   Performing the 40-meter push/walk.

Equipment

This test requires a stopwatch or a watch with a second hand. The test should be conducted on a hard, flat, smooth surface. A starting line is placed 45 meters (49 yards, 8 inches) from a finish line, and a timing line is placed 5 meters (5 yards, 17 inches) from the starting line (figure 5.19). There should also be a safety zone of at least 5 meters beyond the finish line.

Scoring and Trials

Participants are timed to the nearest second over the 40-meter distance. The tester begins timing when the individual crosses the timing line and stops timing when the individual crosses the finish line. As soon as the participant crosses the finish line, the tester measures the participant's radial pulse for 10 seconds. For the correct level of exercise intensity, participants who walk or push a wheelchair with their legs must have a posttest 10-second pulse rate of 20 beats or fewer. Those who push a wheelchair with their arms must have a posttest 10-second pulse rate of 19 beats or fewer. Two trials can be administered if necessary. If two trials are used, permit at least 1 minute of rest between trials. The participant's pulse must be at or near resting level before a trial is administered. The test is assessed on a pass/fail basis. Participants pass when they cover the distance within 60 seconds at the acceptable heart rate intensity.

Test Modifications

If testers experience difficulty with obtaining a radial pulse manually, it is recommended that they use a stethoscope to determine heart rate. Testers can also choose to use a heart rate monitor rather than take a manual radial pulse. If a monitor is used, it should be read within 5 seconds after the individual crosses the finish line. For youngsters who walk or push a wheelchair with their legs, the posttest heart rate on the monitor must be at or below 125 beats per minute. For participants who propel a chair with their arms, the rate must be at or below 115 beats per minute.

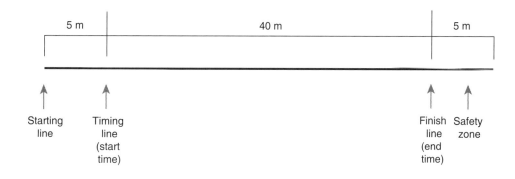

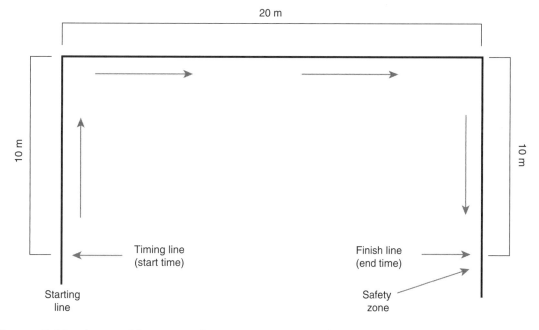

Figure 5.19 Acceptable courses for the 40-meter push/walk.

Suggestions for Test Administration

- If a participant covers the distance in fewer than 60 seconds but the heart rate is too high, provide a rest, instruct the individual to go slower, and retest.

- Testers should not use "on your mark, get set, go" or similar instructions to start the test. Instead, the participant should start from the starting line when he or she is ready, and the tester should begin timing as the participant crosses the timing line.

- Testers can use participants' ratings of perceived exertion or tester observation of exertion to determine below-moderate effort in completing the test (though these procedures are not preferred because they are believed to be less accurate than heart rate measurements). For example, participants who are able to carry on a conversation comfortably or who indicate that the activity was at a "light" exertion level might be considered to have exercised below a moderate level of intensity.

MUSCULOSKELETAL FUNCTIONING: MUSCULAR STRENGTH AND ENDURANCE

Reverse Curl 🎬

In the reverse curl, the participant attempts to pick up a 1-pound (0.5-kilogram) dumbbell with the preferred arm while seated in a chair or wheelchair. The test is designed as a measure of hand, wrist, and arm strength. During the movement, the fingers are flexed (i.e., wrapped around the weight), and the forearm is pronated both at the start and throughout the movement. The movement is executed primarily by extending the wrist and flexing the elbow. It starts with the weight resting on the midpoint of the ipsilateral thigh while the participant is in a normal seated position (figure 5.20a). From this starting position, the participant flexes the elbow and lifts the weight until the elbow is flexed to at least 45 degrees (figure 5.20b). The weight is held in this position for 2 seconds, then returned eccentrically to the starting position. The movement must be controlled, and the elbow extension on the downward movement must be slower than gravitational pull.

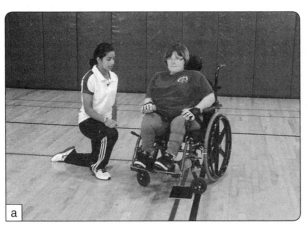 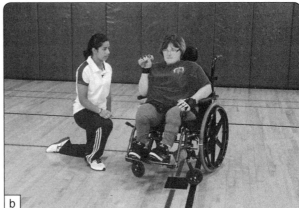

Figure 5.20 Reverse curl: *(a)* starting position and *(b)* up position.

Equipment

The recommended equipment is a 1-pound (0.5-kilogram) soft-iron dumbbell.

Scoring and Trials

One trial is administered. One correct reverse curl involves bringing the dumbbell from the thigh to the flexed-arm position, holding it in the flexed position for 2 seconds, and returning it to the thigh in a controlled manner. The test item is passed if the participant can perform one correct reverse curl.

Test Modifications

- A table or other surface can be used for a starting support surface in place of the thigh. If an alternative support surface is used, it should be at the participant's knee level while seated.
- Weights of 1 pound (0.5 kilogram) other than dumbbells can be used if the testing procedures can be essentially reproduced with them.

Suggestions for Test Administration

- Permit participants to practice the reverse curl before the formal test is administered.
- Provide a positive environment and positive reinforcement of good effort, proper execution, and successful completion of the task.

Seated Push-Up 🎥

In this test, participants attempt to perform a seated push-up and hold it for as long as 20 seconds. The test is designed to measure upper-body strength and endurance. Participants place their hands on the handles of push-up blocks (figure 5.21a), on the armrests of a standard wheelchair or armchair, or on the wheels of a sport wheelchair that does not have armrests (figure 5.21b), and then lift the body so that the buttocks are raised from the supporting surface by extension of the elbows. Once extension is obtained, participants maintain that position for as long as possible; the arms must be extended at the elbow.

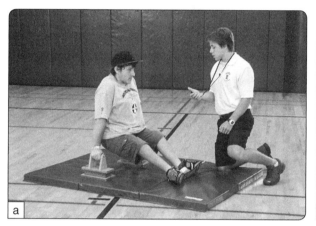
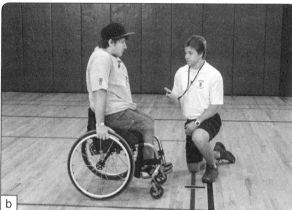

Figure 5.21 Seated push-up performed *(a)* on a mat with push-up blocks and *(b)* on the wheels of a sport wheelchair.

Equipment

This test requires a stopwatch and a standard wheelchair with armrests, a sport wheelchair, a sturdy armchair, or a set of push-up blocks. The armrests (or wheels on a sport wheelchair) or push-up blocks should be slightly more than shoulder-width apart.

Scoring and Trials

The participant performs one trial only. The score is the length of time for which the participant holds the body off of the seat or supporting surface with elbow extension. Feet can come into contact with the floor but cannot be used to assist in performing the push-up. Timing begins when the participant raises the body and obtains elbow extension. Timing ends when the participant no longer holds the position or after a maximum of 20 seconds.

Test Modifications

The test can be administered within the participant's range of motion as long as the buttocks are not in contact with the supporting surface. If the participant is unable to completely extend the elbows due to an impairment, timing should begin when the participant achieves his or her maximal extension and end when the maximal extension is no longer held.

Suggestions for Test Administration

- Take care that participants are in the correct position for testing.
- If using push-up blocks, the tester should stabilize the blocks before the test to prevent them from tipping during the test.
- Give participants an opportunity to practice.

Trunk Lift

In this test item, the participant attempts to lift the upper body as far as 12 inches (30 centimeters) off the floor using muscles of the back and to hold the position to allow for measurement. The test is designed to measure trunk extension, strength, and flexibility. The participant lies on a mat in a prone position (facedown). The toes are pointed, and the hands are placed under the thighs. A coin or other marker may be placed on the mat in line with the participant's eyes. The participant lifts the upper body off the floor to a maximum height of 12 inches (30 centimeters); see figure 5.22. The movement should be performed in a very slow and controlled manner, and the participant should continue to look at the coin or marker throughout the test to enhance correct alignment of the head. The position is held long enough to allow the tester to measure the distance from the participant's chin to the floor. For safety, the ruler should be placed on the floor at least 1 inch (2.5 centimeters) in front of the participant's chin—not directly under the chin. After the tester makes the measurement, the participant returns to the starting position in a controlled manner.

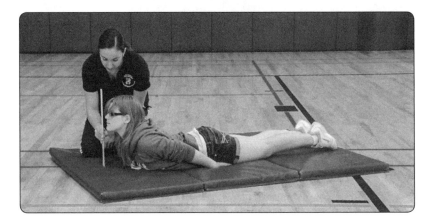

Figure 5.22   Trunk lift.

Equipment

This test requires gym mats and a measuring stick.

Scoring and Trials

Allow two trials and record the better score to the nearest inch or centimeter. Stretches beyond 12 inches (30 centimeters) are discouraged; therefore, scores beyond that distance should be recorded as 12 inches (30 centimeters).

Test Modifications

For persons with intellectual disability, it is permissible to hold the legs in place on the mat during the test. Individuals with disability should be given sufficient time to practice the test and become thoroughly familiar with the testing procedure. When explaining the test item to participants who are blind, it may be helpful to have them feel an individual demonstrating the skill. If the participant cannot see the coin or marker, he or she should be taught to hold the head at a similar angle.

Suggestions for Test Administration

- Do not allow participants to do ballistic (bouncing) movements.
- Do not encourage participants to rise higher than 12 inches (30 centimeters). Excessive arching of the back can cause compression of the disks.
- Because motivation is an important factor, give positive reinforcement continually throughout the test.
- Pay particular attention to performance technique during this test.

Wheelchair Ramp Test

In this test, participants in wheelchairs attempt to push their chairs up a standard wheelchair ramp (figure 5.23). The test is designed to measure upper-body strength and endurance. Participants may use whatever wheelchair push technique they prefer to complete the test.

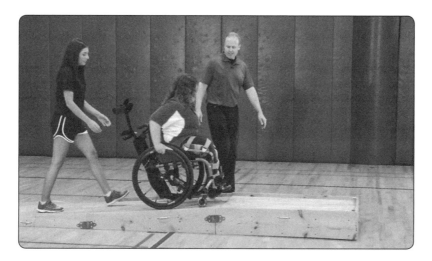

Figure 5.23 Wheelchair ramp test.

Equipment

A standard wheelchair ramp is required. A standard ramp is one that complies with American National Standards Institute (ANSI) guidelines, which specify that ramps should be at least 36 inches (91 centimeters) wide and constructed with 12 inches (30 centimeters) of run for every 1 inch (2.5 centimeters) of rise. For example, a ramp with an elevation of 14 inches (36 centimeters) should be 14 feet (4.3 meters) long. For this test, the ramp must be at least 8 feet (2.4 meters) long. On longer ramps, testers should place lines 8 feet (2.4 meters), 15 feet (4.6 meters), and 30 feet (9.1 meters) from the start of the incline. (Ramps longer than 30 feet generally have a level platform at the 30-foot mark.) It is anticipated that testers will use existing ramps in their schools or buildings to conduct this test, though a ramp with sufficient run is not difficult to construct (see appendix B).

Scoring and Trials

Participants start with their lead wheels off the ramp and attempt to get their rear wheels beyond the lines on the ramp. Going beyond the 8-foot (2.4-meter) line satisfies the minimal standard for this test. The preferred standard is obtained when the individual either goes beyond the 15-foot (4.6-meter) line or makes it to the top of a longer ramp that the individual frequently encounters (e.g., a 20-foot [6.1-meter] ramp leading to the school entrance). Therefore, testers can set a preferred standard between 15 and 30 feet (4.6 and 9.1 meters) based on the typical environment that a participant must negotiate. The test is not timed, and multiple trials are permissible as appropriate.

Test Modifications

The test can be conducted on a ramp that does not meet the ANSI incline standards, provided that it is otherwise safe, but in such cases the tester will have to develop individualized standards.

Suggestions for Test Administration

Safety precautions should be taken to ensure that the wheelchair cannot roll off the edge of the ramp. Participants should be spotted from behind in case the wheelchair begins to roll back down the incline.

Modified Apley Test

The participant attempts to reach back with one hand and touch the superior medial angle of the opposite scapula. The test is designed to measure upper-body flexibility.

Equipment

None.

Scoring and Trials

One trial is given for each arm. If the participant can successfully touch the superior medial angle of the opposite scapula and hold that position for 1 to 2 seconds, a score of 3 is awarded for that arm. If the participant cannot achieve a score of 3, he or she attempts to touch the top of the head; a successful attempt at this target obtains a score of 2. If the participant cannot achieve a score of 2, he or she attempts to touch the mouth and receives a score of 1 if successful. If the participant is unable to touch the mouth, a score of 0 is given for that arm. The scoring scheme is summarized as follows (also see figure 5.24, *a–c*):

3—Touch the superior medial angle of opposite scapula

2—Touch the top of the head

1—Touch the mouth

0—Unable to touch the mouth

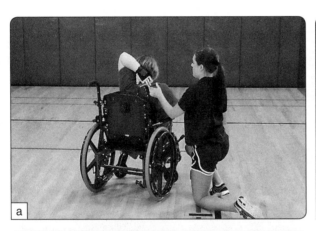

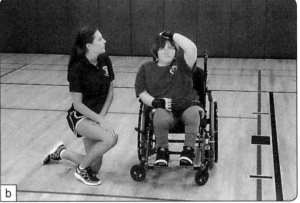

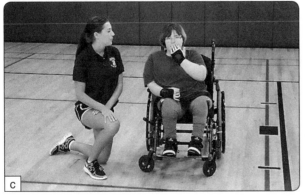

Figure 5.24 Scoring the modified Apley test: *(a)* scapula, score of 3; *(b)* top of head, score of 2; *(c)* mouth, score of 1.

Test Modifications

None.

**MUSCULOSKELETAL FUNCTIONING:
FLEXIBILITY OR RANGE OF MOTION**

Suggestions for Test Administration

- Testers can place their fingertips along the superior medial angle of the scapula (or on the top of the head) to provide a target for the participant and a more objective criterion for scoring (i.e., if the participant can touch the tester's fingertips, a passing score is awarded).
- Participants should be given ample opportunity to practice this test. Physical assistance may be provided during practice but not during the test.
- Participants should be given encouragement and positive reinforcement.
- Testers must require youngsters to hold the test position briefly (1 to 2 seconds) to award a score of 3. Ballistic or reflexive touches are not acceptable.
- Testing should be preceded by sufficient warm-up, including shoulder-stretching activities.

Back-Saver Sit-and-Reach

The objective of this test is to reach across a sit-and-reach box while keeping one leg straight. The test item is designed to measure flexibility of the hamstring muscles. The participant begins the test by removing his or her shoes (very thin footwear is permitted) and sitting down at the test apparatus. One leg is fully extended with the foot flat against the end of the testing instrument. The other knee is bent, with the sole of this foot flat on the floor 2 to 3 inches (5 to 8 centimeters) to the side of the straight knee. The arms are extended forward over the measuring scale with the hands palms down, one on top of the other. The participant reaches directly forward with both hands along the scale four times and holds the position of the fourth reach for at least 1 second (figure 5.25). After that side is measured, the participant switches the position of the legs and reaches again. The participant can allow the bent knee to move to the side if necessary as the body moves by it.

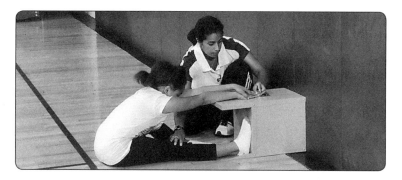

Figure 5.25 Back-saver sit-and-reach.

Equipment

This measurement is best taken using a flexibility testing apparatus approximately 12 inches (30 centimeters) high and 12 inches wide. A measuring scale is placed on top of the apparatus with the zero end of the ruler nearest the participant and the 9-inch (23-centimeter) mark even with the vertical surface against which the foot rests (see appendix B and figures 5.25 and 5.26). The grid on the box should range from 0 to at least 16 inches (41 centimeters).

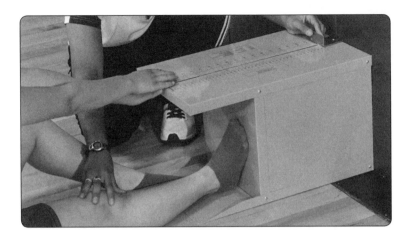

Figure 5.26   Commercially built Flex-Tester.

Scoring and Trials

One trial (four stretches, holding the last) is given for each leg. The tester records, to the nearest whole unit, the number of inches or centimeters reached in the last attempt on each side. Reaches beyond the criterion-referenced standards designated for this test item are not recommended.

Test Modifications

Subjects with intellectual disability should be given sufficient practice time to become completely familiar with the testing procedure. They should not be encouraged to exceed the recommended criterion-referenced standards for this test item.

For blind participants, provide verbal description of the testing environment and procedure. These participants may be given physical assistance as they practice the test and become familiar with the procedure. However, physical assistance may not be given during the test itself.

If a flexibility-testing apparatus is not available, measurements can be obtained with a ruler extended over a bench turned on its side. This approach may be less accurate than use of the recommended testing apparatus.

Suggestions for Test Administration

- The knee of the extended leg must remain straight. The tester should place one hand on the straightened leg to assist proper positioning.
- The participant's hands should reach forward evenly, and the shoulders should be square to the test apparatus.
- Hips must remain square to the box. Do not allow participants to turn their hips away from the box as they reach.
- Require participants to stretch the hamstrings and lower back as a warm-up before testing.
- Because motivation is an important factor, participants should receive continual encouragement and positive reinforcement during the testing process.
- Emphasize a gradual reach forward. Do not permit bobbing or jerking movements forward.

Shoulder Stretch

This test item is used to determine whether a participant is able to touch the fingertips together behind the back by reaching over the shoulder and down the back with one arm and across the back with the other arm (figure 5.27). The test measures upper-body flexibility. The measure is designated *right* or *left* on the basis of the arm reaching over the shoulder; for example, when the right arm stretches over the right shoulder, it is a right-arm stretch.

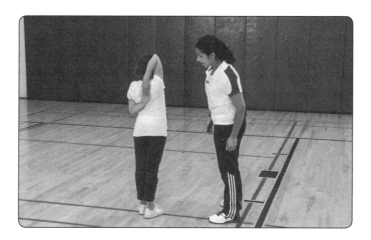

Figure 5.27   Shoulder stretch: right shoulder.

Equipment

None.

Scoring and Trials

One test trial is permitted. The test is scored on a pass/fail basis. The participant passes if the fingers touch and fails if the fingers do not touch.

Test Modifications

Physical assistance and verbal direction may be given to participants as they practice the test. However, physical assistance may not be given during the test itself.

Suggestions for Test Administration

- Participants should be given ample opportunity to practice this testing procedure.
- The recommended warm-up is for upper-body stretching, including approximations of the test itself.

MUSCULOSKELETAL FUNCTIONING: FLEXIBILITY OR RANGE OF MOTION

MUSCULOSKELETAL FUNCTIONING: FLEXIBILITY OR RANGE OF MOTION

Modified Thomas Test

This test is designed to assess the length of the participant's hip flexor muscles. It is conducted on a sturdy table (see figure 5.28, *a–d*). The tester places a thin strip of masking tape on the table 11 inches (28 centimeters) from one of the short edges. The participant lies in a supine position on the table so that the head of the femur is level with the strip of tape. (The tester should ensure that the hip joint is 11 inches from the edge of the table.) The lower legs can be relaxed and should hang off the narrow edge of the table. To test the right hip, the participant lifts the left knee toward the chest. The participant uses the hands to pull the knee toward the chest until the back is flat against the table. At that point, the tester should observe the position of the participant's right thigh. Participants receive the maximum score if they can keep the thigh in contact with the table surface while the back is flat. To test the left hip, the procedure is repeated on the opposite side of the body.

Equipment

This test requires a sturdy table with a tape mark 11 inches (28 centimeters) from one of its short edges. File cards—measuring 3 by 5 inches (i.e., 7.6 centimeters tall) and 4 by 6 inches (15.2 centimeters wide)—or their equivalents are recommended to help with the scoring. A tape measure or ruler can also be used.

Scoring and Trials

One trial for each leg is appropriate for most participants. The test is scored on a scale of 0 to 3 points as follows:

3—The tested leg remains in contact with the surface of the table when the opposite knee is pulled toward the chest, and the back is flat. See figure 5.28*a*.

2—The tested leg does not remain in contact with the surface of the table, but the height of the participant's leg above the edge of the table is less than 3 inches (7.6 centimeters). For example, if the leg is elevated but the tester cannot slide the 3-inch (7.6-centimeter) side of the small file card under the participant's thigh at the edge of the table, a score of 2 is appropriate. See figure 5.28*b*.

1—The tested leg is raised more than 3 inches (7.6 centimeters) but less than 6 inches (15.2 centimeters) above the edge of the table. For example, if the 3-inch (7.6-centimeter) side of the small file card slides under the participant's leg at the edge of the table, but the 6-inch (15.2-centimeter) side of the large card does not, a score of 1 is appropriate. See figure 5.28*c*.

0—The tested leg is raised more than 6 inches (15.2 centimeters) above the edge of the table. For example, if the 6-inch (15.2-centimeter) side of the large file card slides under the participant's thigh at the edge of the table, a score of 0 is appropriate. See figure 5.28*d*.

Test Modifications

If necessary, a tester or spotter can gently assist the participant in pulling the opposite knee toward the chest. In any event, it is important that the back be flat on the table before scoring the test.

If a participant is unable to flatten the lower back after multiple attempts, the tester should score the test as previously indicated and note on the score sheet that the back was not flat. Scores obtained in this manner should not be compared with the standards recommended in this manual. Instead, these scores can be used to monitor future progress, and testers are encouraged to develop individualized standards for the participant.

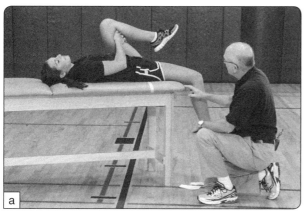
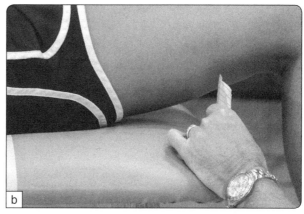
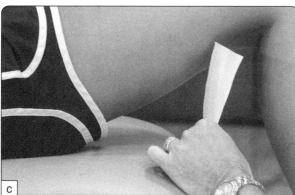
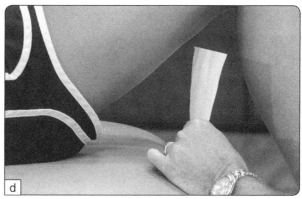

Figure 5.28 Scoring the modified Thomas test: *(a)* score of 3, *(b)* score of 2, *(c)* score of 1, and *(d)* score of 0.

Suggestions for Test Administration

- Participants should stretch or otherwise warm up the hip muscles before testing.
- If testers prefer to use a tape measure or ruler to measure the elevation of the tested leg, the measurement should be taken vertically from the edge of the table to the posterior aspect of the upper leg.
- Testers can determine flatness of the participant's lower back by attempting to pass their hand between the hollow part of the lower back and the table. Ordinarily, the hand is unable to move between the lower back and the table if the back is flat.
- Testers should note any knee extension or thigh abduction that occurs during the test for participants who score a 3. If the rectus femoris extends the knee or the tensor fasciae latae abducts the thigh, some of the hip flexors (iliopsoas and sartorius) are of normal length but others may be shortened.

Target Stretch Test

The target stretch test (TST) is a screening instrument used to estimate movement extent in a joint. It includes a series of tests illustrated in the sketches in form 5.1. For each individual test, testers ask participants to achieve their maximal movement extent for a given joint action and subjectively evaluate that limit against criteria provided in the sketches. Testers should demonstrate or clearly describe the optimal (i.e., complete) movement extent for each joint being tested. The needs of the youngster determine which joints are selected for testing. Individual test items are described in the following entries.

Wrist Extension

The participant's recommended test position is either standing or seated with the elbow flexed to 90 degrees and the forearm pronated (palm down). Participants extend the wrist as far as possible, and testers read the angle made by the longitudinal axis (i.e., lengthwise middle) of the lateral aspect of the hand (not the fingers).

Elbow Extension

The participant's recommended test position is either standing erect or seated with the upper arm at the side. Preferably, the forearm should be supinated (palm facing forward). Participants extend the elbow as far as possible, and testers read the angle made by the longitudinal axis of the forearm from elbow to wrist (not the hand or fingers).

Shoulder Extension

The participant's recommended test position is either standing erect or seated with the arm at the side (palm facing the side). Participants extend the arm backward in a vertical plane as far as the shoulder allows, and testers read the angle made by the longitudinal axis of the upper arm from shoulder to elbow while ensuring that the participant's trunk remains erect.

Shoulder Abduction

The participant's recommended test position is either standing erect or seated with the arm at the side. Participants abduct the shoulder as far as possible, and testers read the angle made by the longitudinal axis of the upper arm from the shoulder to the elbow while ensuring that the participant's trunk remains erect. When the shoulder is fully abducted, the palm should face inward (i.e., toward the midline of the body).

Shoulder External Rotation

The participant's recommended test position is seated so that the tester can evaluate the movement by observing the participant's shoulder from behind and above. The recommended position also requires 90 degrees of elbow flexion and contact between the upper arm and the lateral aspect of the trunk (i.e., adduction). Participants externally rotate the shoulder as far as possible by moving the wrist away from the trunk while maintaining an adducted upper arm and 90 degrees of elbow flexion (see figure 5.29). The tester reads the angle made by the longitudinal axis of the forearm from elbow to wrist from the starting position to the maximum rotated position.

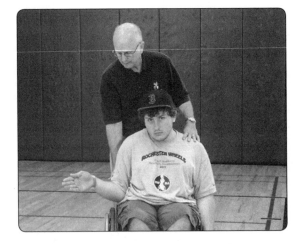

Figure 5.29 Position for the right shoulder external rotation test.

Forearm Supination

The participant's recommended test position is either standing or seated, facing the tester, with elbow flexed while holding a pencil (or similar object) in a closed fist. (The long end of the pencil should protrude up from the thumb side of the fist.) The participant supinates the forearm (palm up) as far as possible, and the tester reads the angle made by the long end of the pencil.

Forearm Pronation

The participant's recommended test position is either standing or seated, facing the tester, with elbow flexed while holding a pencil (or similar object) in a closed fist. (The long end of the pencil should protrude up from the thumb side of the fist.) The participant pronates the forearm (palm down) as far as possible, and the tester reads the angle made by the long end of the pencil.

Knee Extension

The recommended test position is to have the participant in a side-lying position on a rug or mat. (The bottom leg may be bent for stability while the knee of the top leg is being evaluated.) The tester views the extended top leg from above while standing behind the knee being evaluated. The tester reads the angle made by the longitudinal axis of the tested leg from knee to ankle.

Equipment

A firm mat or comfortable rug is helpful for the knee extension test; no other equipment is necessary for participants who are able to achieve the recommended test positions. The tester compares the participant's movements with the criteria provided in the sketches. The test can be administered to participants who cannot achieve the recommended test positions, but evaluation of performance may be enhanced by using a modified goniometer (figure 5.30). Use of this instrument is discussed under test modifications.

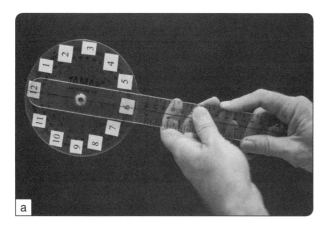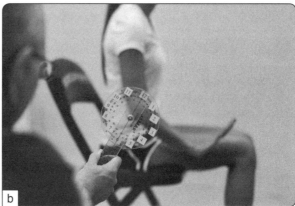

Figure 5.30 Modified goniometer: *(a)* close-up view and *(b)* measuring wrist extension.
Photos courtesy of Matthew J. Yeoman.

Scoring and Trials

Participants must be able to hold their final position for at least 1 second. Using a TST worksheet (form 5.1), testers initially record the "time on the clock" (i.e., the degrees of the arc) of the movement extent to the nearest "half hour" (15 degrees), then convert the "time" to a test score (0 to 2) as given by the sketches. For example, a right wrist extension time of 1:00 receives a score of 2, and times between 1:30 and 2:00 receive a score of 1. Any time below 2:00 receives a score of 0. Noting time on the clock allows the tester to document changes in performance even if the test score does not change. The relationship between test scores and goniometric values is given in table 5.3.

MUSCULOSKELETAL FUNCTIONING: FLEXIBILITY OR RANGE OF MOTION

Table 5.3 Goniometric Values Associated With Target Stretch Test Scores

	Normal[a]	2	1
Wrist extension	70°	60°	30°
Elbow extension	0°	0°	–15°
Shoulder extension	60°	60°	30°
Shoulder abduction	170°	165°	120°
Shoulder external rotation	90°	75°	30°
Supination/pronation	90°	90°	45°
Knee extension	0°	0°	–15°

[a] Normal, or typical, range-of-motion values found in the literature vary somewhat from authority to authority. These values come from Cole and Tobis (1990). In some cases, values for test scores of 2 differ from Cole and Tobis's values due to the recommendation that testers estimate movement extent to the nearest "half hour" (15°). In the case of shoulder external rotation, part of the difference between a normal score and a score of 2 involves differences in test procedures.

Adapted from Cole and Tobis, 1990.

Form 5.1　Target Stretch Test

a) Wrist extension (left)

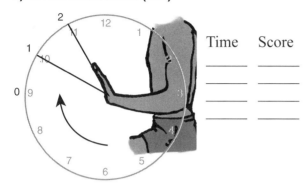

Time　Score

_____　_____
_____　_____
_____　_____
_____　_____

Position _____

Comments _____

b) Wrist extension (right)

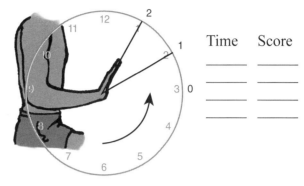

Time　Score

_____　_____
_____　_____
_____　_____
_____　_____

Position _____

Comments _____

c) Elbow extension (left)

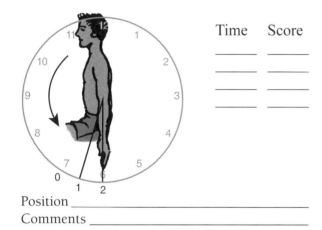

Time　Score

_____　_____
_____　_____
_____　_____

Position _____

Comments _____

d) Elbow extension (right)

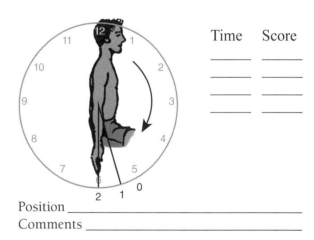

Time　Score

_____　_____
_____　_____
_____　_____
_____　_____

Position _____

Comments _____

e) Shoulder extension (left)

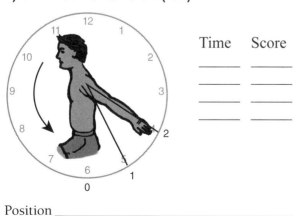

Time　Score

_____　_____
_____　_____
_____　_____
_____　_____

Position _____

Comments _____

f) Shoulder extension (right)

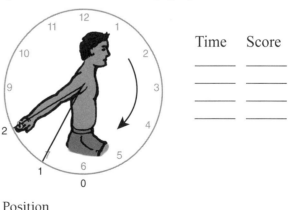

Time　Score

_____　_____
_____　_____
_____　_____
_____　_____

Position _____

Comments _____

(continued)

g) Shoulder abduction (left)

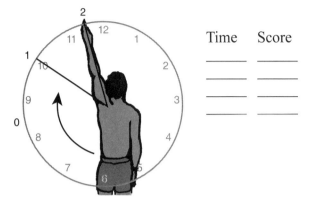

Time   Score

_____   _____
_____   _____
_____   _____
_____   _____

Position _____
Comments _____

h) Shoulder abduction (right)

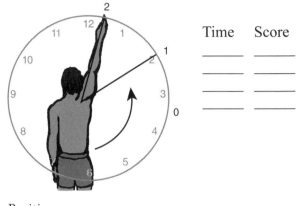

Time   Score

_____   _____
_____   _____
_____   _____
_____   _____

Position _____
Comments _____

i) Shoulder external rotation (left)

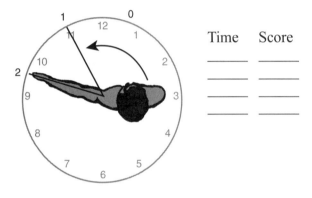

Time   Score

_____   _____
_____   _____
_____   _____
_____   _____

Position _____
Comments _____

j) Shoulder external rotation (right)

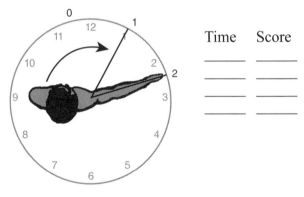

Time   Score

_____   _____
_____   _____
_____   _____
_____   _____

Position _____
Comments _____

k) Forearm supination (left)

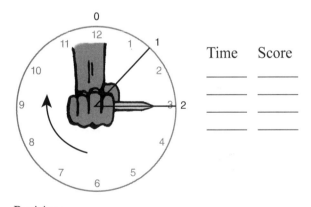

Time   Score

_____   _____
_____   _____
_____   _____
_____   _____

Position _____
Comments _____

l) Forearm supination (right)

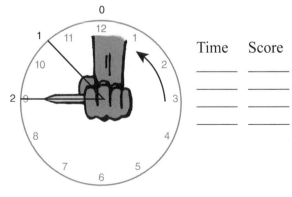

Time   Score

_____   _____
_____   _____
_____   _____
_____   _____

Position _____
Comments _____

m) Forearm pronation (left)

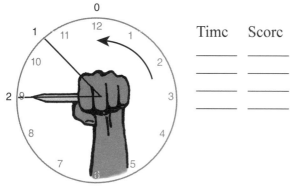

Time	Score
_____	_____
_____	_____
_____	_____
_____	_____

Position _____

Comments _____

n) Forearm pronation (right)

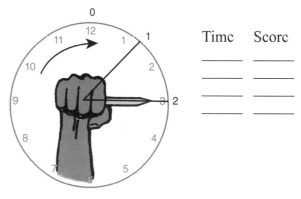

Time	Score
_____	_____
_____	_____
_____	_____
_____	_____

Position _____

Comments _____

o) Knee extension (left)

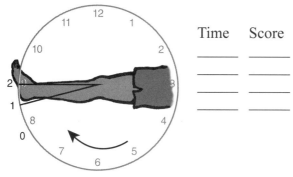

Time	Score
_____	_____
_____	_____
_____	_____
_____	_____

Position _____

Comments _____

p) Knee extension (right)

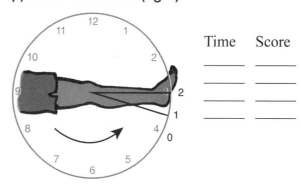

Time	Score
_____	_____
_____	_____
_____	_____
_____	_____

Position _____

Comments _____

From J. Winnick and F. Short, 2014, *Brockport physical fitness test manual: A health-related assessment for youngsters with disabilities* (Champaign, IL: Human Kinetics).

Test Modifications

If a participant cannot achieve the recommended test position depicted in the sketch, the joint action can still be assessed, but the clock must be rotated for scoring. For instance, the recommended test position for right wrist extension includes maintaining elbow flexion of 90 degrees. A participant could, however, be tested with the arm at the side and a completely extended elbow if the clock is rotated 90 degrees so that the 9 instead of the 12 is at the top of the clock. This approach may become conceptually difficult for the tester, so it is recommended that testers modify a transparent plastic goniometer to help rotate the clock into the proper position. The circular dial of the goniometer can be converted into a version of a clock face by placing the numerals 1 to 12 on strips of tape at 30-degree intervals (figure 5.30a). Once the goniometer is modified, it can be used to rotate the clock and estimate movement extent from a variety of test positions. When using the modified goniometer, it is recommended that testers stand, crouch, or kneel approximately 5 to 10 feet (about 1.5 to 3 meters) from the participant. The tester reads the time on the clock by holding the goniometer at arm's length and viewing the limb in question through the face of the goniometer (figure 5.30b).

Testers who are knowledgeable about and comfortable with taking actual goniometry measures may prefer that approach to estimating movement extent via the clock. Test scores of 0, 1, and 2 can be assigned based on the goniometric values given in table 5.3.

Suggestions for Test Administration

- Testers should help participants maximize their movement extent. Changes in body position may influence a participant's performance. Youngsters who have tonic neck reflexes, for instance, may enhance their performance by flexing, extending, or turning the head while being tested. Testers should help participants find the position that maximizes the movement extent in a joint, as long as the position is noted on the worksheet and the integrity of the scoring system is maintained (e.g., the clock may need to be rotated).

- When evaluating a number of participants, testers can expedite the process by recording the movement extent on the clock during testing and converting it to a score after the testing session.

- Participants should warm up the joints to be tested.

- Testers may find it helpful to tape photocopies of the sketches (enlargements work best) to a nearby wall in order to eliminate flipping back and forth between pages in the manual or worksheet.

- Testers who administer the TST may find the worksheet in form 5.1 helpful and are free to photocopy it as often as necessary. The sketches demonstrate the recommended test positions, the clock for scoring, and the criteria for both specific standards (a score of 1) and general standards (a score of 2). Spaces are available to the right of each sketch to record both time on the clock (degree of movement) to the nearest half hour and corresponding test score (0 to 2). Extra space is provided to allow multiple administrations of the test. Below each sketch, room is given to note any variation in test position that is necessary when a participant cannot attain the recommended test position. There is also room to note other relevant observations.

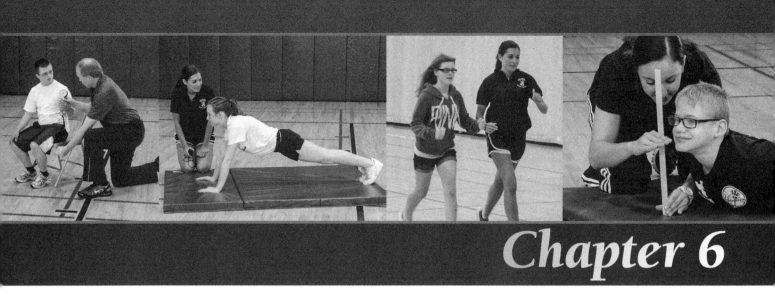

Chapter 6

Testing Youngsters With Severe Disability

The Brockport Physical Fitness Test (BPFT) is appropriate for many youngsters with disability and unique needs related to physical fitness. However, it may be inappropriate for youngsters with severe disability for a variety of reasons. Often, these reasons include the inability of such students to perform field-based performance test items as described in the procedures presented in this manual. Specifically, these individuals may lack the level of physical fitness, motivation, understanding, or basic motor ability required to perform test items.

For such individuals, two alternative orientations for assessment are offered in this chapter. These orientations may yield information about physical activity or physical fitness and may most appropriately serve as the basis for individualized rather than health-related, criterion-referenced standards. However, their results may be helpful in designing programs that lead to acceptable levels of physical fitness or physical activity. The two orientations are alternate assessment and measurement of physical activity.

Alternate Assessment

Two types of alternate assessment recommended for youngsters with severe disability are task

analysis and rubrics. Task analysis breaks movements, skills, and activities into tasks and possibly subtasks. Tasks are associated with outcomes that can be targeted, learned, and measured. They represent points of focus in the performance of an activity. Ideally, they take an individual from a present level of performance through activities leading to a terminal objective. Task analyses can be designed in a variety of ways.

Using task analysis to develop and assess physical fitness in people with severe disability is not new. Jansma, Decker, Ersing, McCubbin, and Combs (1988) presented the Project Transition assessment system and contrasted it with the Data Based Gymnasium, I CAN, and Project MOBILITEE models. Readers are also referred to curriculum materials developed in connection with adapted sport programs.

In recent years, the field of adapted physical education has emphasized the use of ecological task analysis to best meet the measurement and instructional needs of students. Ecological task analysis considers the components of a skill or activity (traditional task analysis), as well as students' limitations and capabilities and the environment. For in-depth information about both traditional and ecological task analysis, see Winnick (2011).

A second alternative approach for assessing physical fitness is the use of rubrics, which are essentially rating scales wherein characteristics describing performance are matched to selected points on a scale. Although rubrics often lack the psychometric qualities associated with standardized tests, they lend themselves well to individualized assessment and can be designed to measure abilities at various points on an achievement continuum. Rubrics have also been called rating scales, scoring rubrics, analytic rating scales, and checklists. Detailed information about the development of rubrics is available in books addressing the teaching and assessment of physical education and adapted physical education.

Task analysis and rubrics are recommended in this manual for the purpose of leading youngsters toward acceptable levels of health-related physical fitness. Figure 6.1 and table 6.1 provide a sample task analysis and a sample rubric, respectively, for the isometric push-up test item of the BPFT.

Measurement of Physical Activity

Before procedures are recommended for measuring physical activity, it is important to remember that physical activity and physical fitness are separate but related concepts. Measurement of physical *fitness* involves measuring characteristics reflecting abilities that people possess or develop. The BPFT is used to measure physical fitness. Measurement of physical *activity* typically involves measuring a behavior reflecting energy expenditure. Examples of physical activity measures include heart rate responses to exercise; caloric expenditure; and the frequency, intensity, type, and duration of activity.

Measurements of physical activity can be attained or estimated using a variety of strategies, including direct observation, self-report measures, mechanical and electronic monitoring, and physiological measures. These strategies are presented and discussed in a variety of sources (e.g., Freedson & Melanson, 1996; Welk & Wood, 2000). Devices that appear to hold promise for obtaining accurate measurements of physical activity in individuals with severe disability include pedometers, accelerometers, motion sensors, and heart rate monitors.

Teachers are encouraged to monitor the frequency, intensity, type, and duration of physical activity in youngsters with more severe disabilities and to develop strategies for increasing those levels. The Activitygram developed by the Cooper Institute (2010) is an effective computer-assisted tool for measuring and assessing the physical activity of children. It uses a physical activity recall approach for data collection. Increases in physical activity often lead to increases in physical fitness, even if fitness is difficult to assess validly.

Because physical fitness and physical activity may have independent effects on health status (Blair, Kohl, Paffenbarger, Clark, Cooper, & Gibbons, 1990), different standards may also be needed and recommended for each. The U.S. Department of Health and Human Services (2008) recommends that children and adolescents do 60 minutes or more of daily physical activity, which should include aerobic, muscle-strengthening, and bone-strengthening activities. The agency encourages participation in activities that are age appropriate, enjoyable, and varied.

Sample Task Analysis for an Isometric Push-Up

Objective

To execute an isometric push-up correctly for 3 seconds.

Directions

Circle the minimal level of assistance an individual requires when correctly performing a task. Total each column. Total the column scores and enter the total score in the summary section. Determine the score for percentage of independence by dividing the scores achieved by the possible scores. For the product score, record the amount of time for which the position is held.

Isometric push-up	IND	PPA	TPA
1. Lie facedown.	(3)	2	1
2. Place hands under shoulders.	(3)	2	1
3. Place legs straight, slightly apart, and parallel to the floor.	3	(2)	1
4. Tuck toes under feet.	3	(2)	1
5. Extend arms while body is in a straight line.	3	2	(1)
6. Hold position for 3 seconds.	3	2	(1)
Sum of column scores	6	4	2

Key to levels of assistance:
  IND = independent (able to perform the task without assistance)
  PPA = partial physical assistance (needs some assistance to perform the task)
  TPA = total physical assistance (needs total assistance to perform the task)			

SUMMARY			
Total score achieved	12		
Total score possible	18		
% independent score	67		
Product score (position held)	3 seconds		

Adapted, by permission, from L.J. Lieberman and C. Houston-Wilson, 2009, *Strategies for inclusion: A handbook for physical educators*, 2nd ed. (Champaign, IL: Human Kinetics), 35.

Figure 6.1 Sample task analysis.

Table 6.1 Rubric for Isometric Push-Up

Level of performance	Characteristic behaviors
Mastery	Can perform the isometric push-up with proper mechanics and is able to hold without assistance for 25 seconds
Intermediate	Can perform the isometric push-up without physical assistance for 15 seconds
Intermediate/beginner	Can perform the isometric push-up with some physical assistance for 5 seconds
Beginner	Can perform the correct position with physical assistance for 3 seconds

Appendix A

Body Mass Index (BMI) Chart

This chart provides BMI values for males and females in the general population. To interpret the numbers found in this chart, please refer to the tables presented in chapter 4. Fitness Zone tables 1 and 2 provide BMI interpretation for boys and girls in the general population. Fitness Zone tables 3 through 12 provide BMI interpretation or percent body fat for boys and girls with specific disabilities.

Height (in.) Weight (lb.)	49	51	53	55	57	59	61	63	65	67	69	71	73	75	77	79	81	83
66	19	18	16	15	14	13	12	12	11	10	10	9	9	8	8	8	7	7
70	20	19	18	16	15	14	13	13	12	11	10	10	9	9	8	8	8	7
75	22	20	19	17	16	15	14	13	12	12	11	10	10	9	9	9	8	8
79	23	21	20	18	17	16	15	14	13	12	12	11	11	10	9	9	9	8
84	24	22	21	19	18	17	16	15	14	13	12	12	11	11	10	10	9	9
88	26	24	22	20	19	18	17	16	15	14	13	12	12	11	11	10	10	9
92	27	25	23	21	20	19	17	16	15	15	14	13	12	12	11	11	10	10
97	28	26	24	22	21	20	18	17	16	15	14	14	13	12	12	11	10	10
101	29	27	25	23	22	20	19	18	17	16	15	14	13	13	12	12	11	10
106	31	28	26	24	23	21	20	19	18	17	16	15	14	13	13	12	11	11
110	32	30	27	26	24	22	21	20	18	17	16	15	15	14	13	13	11	11
114	33	31	29	27	25	23	22	20	19	18	17	16	15	14	14	13	12	12
119	35	32	30	28	26	24	22	21	20	19	18	17	16	15	14	14	13	12
123	36	33	31	29	27	25	23	22	21	19	18	17	16	16	15	14	13	13
128	37	34	32	30	28	26	24	23	21	20	19	18	17	16	15	15	14	13
132	38	36	33	31	29	27	25	23	22	21	20	19	18	17	16	15	14	14
136	40	37	34	32	29	28	26	24	23	21	20	19	18	17	16	16	15	14
141	41	38	35	33	30	28	27	25	24	22	21	20	19	18	17	16	15	15
145	42	39	36	34	31	29	27	26	24	23	22	20	19	18	17	17	16	15
150	44	40	37	35	32	30	28	27	25	24	22	21	20	19	18	17	16	15
154	45	41	38	36	33	31	29	27	26	24	23	22	20	19	18	18	17	16
158	46	43	40	37	34	32	30	28	26	25	24	22	21	20	19	18	17	16
163	47	44	41	38	35	33	31	29	27	26	24	23	22	20	19	19	18	17
167	49	45	42	39	36	34	32	30	28	26	25	23	22	21	20	19	18	17
172	50	46	43	40	37	35	32	30	29	27	25	24	23	22	21	20	19	18
176	51	47	44	41	38	36	33	31	29	28	26	25	23	22	21	20	19	18
180	52	49	45	42	39	36	34	32	30	28	27	25	24	23	22	21	20	19
185	54	50	46	43	40	37	35	33	31	29	27	26	25	23	22	21	20	19
189	55	51	47	44	41	38	36	34	32	30	28	27	25	24	23	22	20	20
194	56	52	48	45	42	39	37	34	32	30	29	27	26	24	23	22	21	20
198	58	53	49	46	43	40	37	35	33	31	29	28	26	25	24	23	21	20
202	59	54	50	47	44	41	38	36	34	32	30	28	27	25	24	23	22	21
207	60	56	52	48	45	42	39	37	35	33	31	29	27	26	25	24	22	21
211	61	57	53	49	46	43	40	38	35	33	31	30	28	27	25	24	23	22
216	63	58	54	50	47	44	41	38	36	34	32	30	29	27	26	25	23	22
220	64	59	55	51	48	44	42	39	37	35	33	31	29	28	26	25	24	23
224	65	60	56	52	49	45	42	40	37	35	33	31	30	28	27	26	24	23
229	67	62	57	53	49	46	43	41	38	36	34	32	30	29	27	26	25	24
233	68	63	58	54	50	47	44	41	39	37	35	33	31	29	28	27	25	24
238	69	64	59	55	51	48	45	42	40	37	35	33	32	30	28	27	26	24
242	70	65	60	56	52	49	46	43	40	38	36	34	32	30	29	28	26	25
246	72	66	61	57	53	50	47	44	41	39	37	35	33	31	29	28	27	25
251	73	67	63	58	54	51	47	45	42	39	37	35	33	32	30	29	27	26
255	74	69	64	59	55	52	48	45	43	40	38	36	34	32	31	29	28	26
260	76	70	65	60	56	52	49	46	43	41	39	36	34	33	31	30	28	27
264	77	71	66	61	57	53	50	47	44	42	39	37	35	33	32	30	29	27
268	78	72	67	62	58	54	51	48	45	42	40	38	36	34	32	31	29	28
273	79	73	68	63	59	55	52	48	46	43	40	38	36	34	33	31	30	28
277	81	75	69	64	60	56	52	49	46	44	41	39	37	35	33	32	30	29
282	82	76	70	65	61	57	53	50	47	44	42	40	37	35	34	32	30	29
286	83	77	71	66	62	58	54	51	48	45	42	40	38	36	34	33	31	29
290	84	78	72	67	63	59	55	52	48	46	43	41	39	37	35	33	31	30
295	86	79	74	68	64	60	56	52	49	46	44	41	39	37	35	34	32	30
299	87	80	75	69	65	60	57	53	50	47	44	42	40	38	36	34	32	31
304	88	82	76	70	66	61	57	54	51	48	45	43	40	38	36	35	33	31
308	90	83	77	71	67	62	58	55	51	48	46	43	41	39	37	35	33	32
312	91	84	78	72	68	63	59	55	52	49	46	44	41	39	37	36	34	32

Panel on Energy, Obesity, and Body Weight Standards, 1987, *American Journal of Clinical Nutrition Supplement* 45(5): 1035–1047.

Appendix B

Purchasing and Constructing Unique Testing Supplies

Resources for selected test supplies, page 108

Equipment and construction steps for back-saver sit-and-reach apparatus, page 109

Alternative flexibility-testing apparatuses, page 110

Equipment and construction steps for ramp, page 111

Equipment and construction steps for modified pull-up stand, page 113

Resources for Selected Test Supplies

Test item	Supply item	Resource address	Phone and web contact
Back-saver sit-and-reach	Sit-and-reach apparatus	GOPHER Sport 2525 Lemond St. SW PO Box 998 Owatonna, MN 55060-0998	800-533-0446 www.gophersport.com
Curl-up	Curl-up measuring strips	Human Kinetics PO Box 5076 Champaign, IL 61825-5076	800-747-4457 www.humankinetics.com
Dominant grip strength	Jamar grip dynamometer	Patterson Medical 28100 Torch Parkway Suite 700 Warrenville, IL 60555-3938	800-323-5547 www.pattersonmedical.com
PACER	PACER recording	Human Kinetics PO Box 5076 Champaign, IL 61825-5076	800-747-4457 www.humankinetics.com
Seated push-up	Push-up blocks	Patterson Medical 28100 Torch Parkway Suite 700 Warrenville, IL 60555-3938	800-323-5547 www.pattersonmedical.com
Skinfold test	Skinfold caliper	U.S. Chemical 316 Hart Street Watertown, WI 53094	800-858-2382 http://uschemical.com/beta
Target aerobic movement test (TAMT)	Electronic heart rate monitor (many types available)	GOPHER Sport 2525 Lemond St. SW PO Box 998 Owatonna, MN 55060-0998	800-533-0446 www.gophersport.com

Equipment and Construction Steps
for Back-Saver Sit-and-Reach Apparatus

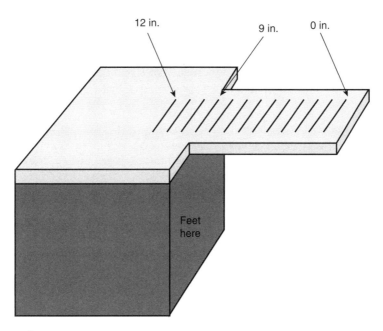

Back-saver sit-and-reach apparatus.

1. Using any sturdy wood or comparable material (3/4-inch [2-centimeter] plywood works well), cut the following pieces:

   Two pieces, 12 inches by 12 inches (30 centimeters by 30 centimeters)

   Two pieces, 12 inches by 10.5 inches (30 centimeters by 26 centimeters)

   One piece, 12 inches by 22 inches (30 centimeters by 56 centimeters)

2. From each corner of one end of the piece measuring 12 inches by 22 inches (30 centimeters by 56 centimeters), cut pieces that are 10 inches by 4 inches (26 centimeters by 10 centimeters) to make the top of the box. Beginning at the small end, make marks on the piece at every inch (or centimeter) up to 12 inches (30 centimeters).

3. Using the four remaining pieces, construct a box secured with nails, screws, or wood glue. Attach the top of the box. The 9-inch (23-centimeter) mark must be exactly in line with the vertical plane against which the participant's foot will be placed. The zero mark is at the end that will be nearest to the participant.

4. Cover the apparatus with polyurethane sealer or shellac.

Adapted, by permission, from The Cooper Institute, 2013, *Fitnessgram/Activitygram test administration manual,* updated 4th ed. (Champaign, IL: Human Kinetics), 88.

Alternative Flexibility-Testing Apparatuses

1. Find a sturdy cardboard box at least 12 inches (30 centimeters) tall. Turn the box so that the bottom is up. Tape a ruler or yardstick (or meter stick) to the bottom. The measuring stick must be placed so that the 9-inch (23-centimeter) mark is exactly in line with the vertical plane against which the participant's foot will be placed and the zero is nearer the participant.

2. Find a bench that is about 12 inches (30 centimeters) wide. Turn the bench on its side. Tape a ruler or yardstick (or meter stick) to the bench so that the 9-inch (23-centimeter) mark is exactly in line with the vertical plane against which the participant's foot will be placed and the zero end is nearer the participant.

Adapted, by permission, from The Cooper Institute, 2013, *Fitnessgram/Activitygram test administration manual*, updated 4th ed. (Champaign, IL: Human Kinetics), 88.

Equipment and Construction Steps for Ramp

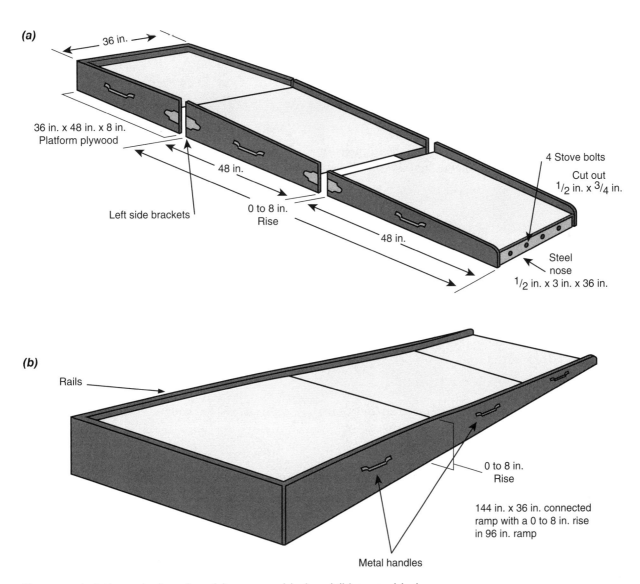

Ramp and platform design plan: *(a)* unassembled and *(b)* assembled.

Reprinted, by permission, from The Cooper Institute, 2010, *The Prudential Fitnessgram test administration manual* (Dallas, TX: The Cooper Institute).

Items Needed

Ramp

One piece of ramp plywood, 3/4 inch by 36 inches by 96 inches (2 centimeters by 91 centimeters by 244 centimeters)

One piece of platform plywood, 3/4 inch by 36 inches by 48 inches (2 centimeters by 91 centimeters by 122 centimeters)

One steel nosing, 1/2 inch by 3 inches by 36 inches (2 centimeters by 8 centimeters by 91 centimeters)

Nails, wood screws, stove bolts

Ramp Supports

Three pieces of wood for ramp plywood, 2 inches by (dimensions ranging from 0 inch to 7 1/2 inches) by 96 inches (5 centimeters by 19 centimeters by 244 centimeters)

One piece of wood for platform plywood, 2 inches by 7 1/2 inches by 33 inches (5 centimeters by 19 centimeters by 83.8 centimeters)

One piece of wood for platform plywood 2 inches by 3 3/4 inches by 33 inches (5 centimeters by 6.25 centimeters by 83.8 centimeters)

Rails

Two pieces of wood for ramp, 1 inch by (dimensions ranging from 2 inches to 10 inches) by 96 inches (2.5 centimeters by 25 centimeters by 244 centimeters)

One piece of wood for platform, 1 inch by 10 inches by 48 inches (2.5 centimeters by 25 centimeters by 122 centimeters)

One piece of wood for platform, 1 inch by 10 inches by 36 inches (2.5 centimeters by 25 centimeters by 91 centimeters)

Handles and Brackets

Six 3 1/2-inch (9-centimeter) metal handles

Two pairs of left-hand brackets

Two pairs of right-hand brackets

Procedure

1. Cut out 1/2 inch (1.3 centimeter) deep by 3/4 inch (2 centimeters) back along the width of one end of the ramp plywood for steel nosing.

2. Drill four holes in plywood and steel nosing.

3. Apply steel nosing using four stove bolts.

4. Assemble ramp in one piece using 2-inch by (dimensions ranging from 0-inch to 7 1/2-inch) by 96-inch (0-centimeter by 19-centimeter by 244-centimeter) base supports running lengthwise under plywood and spaced 18 inches (45 centimeters) apart. Apply 3/4-inch by 36-inch by 96-inch (2-centimeter by 91-centimeter by 244-centimeter) ramp plywood over lengthwise supports using wood screws.

5. Assemble platform in the same way.

6. Cut ramp at 48 inches (122 centimeters) into two sections.

7. Apply 1-inch by (dimensions ranging from 2-inch to 10-inch) by 96-inch (5-centimeter by 25-centimeter by 244-centimeter) rails to sides of ramp after they have been cut in two to fit the dimensions of the ramp plywood.

8. Apply 1-inch by 10-inch by 48-inch (2.5-centimeter by 25-centimeter by 122-centimeter) and 1-inch by 10-inch by 36-inch (2.5-centimeter by 25-centimeter by 91-centimeter) rails to platform.

9. Apply two pairs of left-hand brackets and then two pairs of right-hand brackets to ramp. Brackets overlap to connect.

10. Apply a metal handle to the side of each platform and ramp section.

Reprinted, by permission, from The Cooper Institute, 2010, *The Prudential Fitnessgram test administration manual* (Dallas, TX: The Cooper Institute).

Equipment and Construction Steps
for Modified Pull-Up Stand

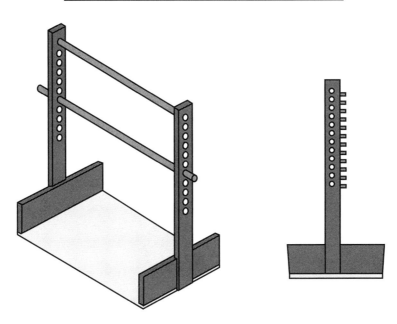

Modified pull-up stand.

Items Needed

One piece of plywood, 3/4 inch by 24 inches by 39 inches (2 centimeters by 61 centimeters by 99 centimeters) for support platform

Two pieces for base of uprights, 2 inches by 8 inches by 24 inches (5 centimeters by 20 centimeters by 61 centimeters)

Two pieces for uprights, 2 inches by 4 inches by 48 inches (5 centimeters by 10 centimeters by 122 centimeters)

One 1 1/8-inch (3 5/8-centimeter) steel pipe for chin-up bar

One 1 1/4-inch (3-centimeter) dowel for top support

Twenty-four 3/8-inch (1-centimeter) dowel pieces cut 3 1/2 inches (9 centimeters) long

Nails, wood screws, and wood glue for construction

Procedure

1. At a point 2 1/2 inches (6.35 centimeters) from the top end of each of the 2-inch by 4-inch by 48-inch (5-centimeter by 10-centimeter by 122-centimeter) pieces, drill a hole through the 2-inch (5-centimeter) width for the 1 1/4-inch (3.625-centimeter) dowel support rod.

2. Below the first hole, drill eleven 1 1/8-inch (3.625-centimeter) holes for the steel pipe. Measure 2 1/2 inches (6.35 centimeters) between the centers of these holes.

3. Beginning 3 3/4 inches (9 5/8 centimeters) from the top of these upright pieces, drill twelve 3/8-inch (1-centimeter) holes into the 4-inch (10-centimeter) width. Center these holes between the holes for the steel pipe.

4. Assemble the pieces and finish with polyurethane or shellac.

Adapted, by permission, from The Cooper Institute, 2013, *Fitnessgram/Activitygram test administration manual,* updated 4th ed. (Champaign, IL: Human Kinetics), 87.

Appendix C

Fitnessgram Body Composition Conversion Charts

BOYS (TRICEPS PLUS CALF SKINFOLD TO % FAT)											
Total mm	% fat	Total mm	% fat	Total mm	% fat	Total mm	% fat	Total mm	% fat	Total mm	% fat
1.0	1.7	16.0	12.8	31.0	23.8	46.0	34.8	61.0	45.8		
1.5	2.1	16.5	13.1	31.5	24.2	46.5	35.2	61.5	46.2		
2.0	2.5	17.0	13.5	32.0	24.5	47.0	35.5	62.0	46.6		
2.5	2.8	17.5	13.9	32.5	24.9	47.5	35.9	62.5	46.9		
3.0	3.2	18.0	14.2	33.0	25.3	48.0	36.3	63.0	47.3		
3.5	3.6	18.5	14.6	33.5	25.6	48.5	36.6	63.5	47.7		
4.0	3.9	19.0	15.0	34.0	26.0	49.0	37.0	64.0	48.0		
4.5	4.3	19.5	15.3	34.5	26.4	49.5	37.4	64.5	48.4		
5.0	4.7	20.0	15.7	35.0	26.7	50.0	37.8	65.0	48.8		
5.5	5.0	20.5	16.1	35.5	27.1	50.5	38.1	65.5	49.1		
6.0	5.4	21.0	16.4	36.0	27.5	51.0	38.5	66.0	49.5		
6.5	5.8	21.5	16.8	36.5	27.8	51.5	38.9	66.5	49.9		
7.0	6.1	22.0	17.2	37.0	28.2	52.0	39.2	67.0	50.2		
7.5	6.5	22.5	17.5	37.5	28.6	52.5	39.6	67.5	50.6		
8.0	6.9	23.0	17.9	38.0	28.9	53.0	40.0	68.0	51.0		
8.5	7.2	23.5	18.3	38.5	29.3	53.5	40.3	68.5	51.3		
9.0	7.6	24.0	18.6	39.0	29.7	54.0	40.7	69.0	51.7		
9.5	8.0	24.5	19.0	39.5	30.0	54.5	41.1	69.5	52.1		
10.0	8.4	25.0	19.4	40.0	30.4	55.0	41.4	70.0	52.5		
10.5	8.7	25.5	19.7	40.5	30.8	55.5	41.8	70.5	52.8		
11.0	9.1	26.0	20.1	41.0	31.1	56.0	42.2	71.0	53.2		
11.5	9.5	26.5	20.5	41.5	31.5	56.5	42.5	71.5	53.6		
12.0	9.8	27.0	20.8	42.0	31.9	57.0	42.9	72.0	53.9		
12.5	10.2	27.5	21.2	42.5	32.2	57.5	43.3	72.5	54.3		
13.0	10.6	28.0	21.6	43.0	32.6	58.0	43.6	73.0	54.7		
13.5	10.9	28.5	21.9	43.5	33.0	58.5	44.0	73.5	55.0		
14.0	11.3	29.0	22.3	44.0	33.3	59.0	44.4	74.0	55.4		
14.5	11.7	29.5	22.7	44.5	33.7	59.5	44.7	74.5	55.8		
15.0	12.0	30.0	23.1	45.0	34.1	60.0	45.1	75.0	56.1		
15.5	12.4	30.5	23.4	45.5	34.4	60.5	45.5	75.5	56.5		

Reprinted, by permission, from The Cooper Institute, 2013, *Fitnessgram/Activitygram test administration manual,* updated 4th ed. (Champaign, IL: Human Kinetics), 101.

\multicolumn{12}{c}{GIRLS (TRICEPS PLUS CALF SKINFOLD TO % FAT)}

Total mm	% fat	Total mm	% fat	Total mm	% fat	Total mm	% fat	Total mm	% fat
1.0	5.7	16.0	14.9	31.0	24.0	46.0	33.2	61.0	42.3
1.5	6.0	16.5	15.2	31.5	24.3	46.5	33.5	61.5	42.6
2.0	6.3	17.0	15.5	32.0	24.6	47.0	33.8	62.0	42.9
2.5	6.6	17.5	15.8	32.5	24.9	47.5	34.1	62.5	43.2
3.0	6.9	18.0	16.1	33.0	25.2	48.0	34.4	63.0	43.5
3.5	7.2	18.5	16.4	33.5	25.5	48.5	34.7	63.5	43.8
4.0	7.5	19.0	16.7	34.0	25.8	49.0	35.0	64.0	44.1
4.5	7.8	19.5	17.0	34.5	26.1	49.5	35.3	64.5	44.4
5.0	8.2	20.0	17.3	35.0	26.5	50.0	35.6	65.0	44.8
5.5	8.5	20.5	17.6	35.5	26.8	50.5	35.9	65.5	45.1
6.0	8.8	21.0	17.9	36.0	27.1	51.0	36.2	66.0	45.4
6.5	9.1	21.5	18.2	36.5	27.4	51.5	36.5	66.5	45.7
7.0	9.4	22.0	18.5	37.0	27.7	52.0	36.8	67.0	46.0
7.5	9.7	22.5	18.8	37.5	28.0	52.5	37.1	67.5	46.3
8.0	10.0	23.0	19.1	38.0	28.3	53.0	37.4	68.0	46.6
8.5	10.3	23.5	19.4	38.5	28.6	53.5	37.7	68.5	46.9
9.0	10.6	24.0	19.7	39.0	28.9	54.0	38.0	69.0	47.2
9.5	10.9	24.5	20.0	39.5	29.2	54.5	38.3	69.5	47.5
10.0	11.2	25.0	20.4	40.0	29.5	55.0	38.7	70.0	47.8
10.5	11.5	25.5	20.7	40.5	29.8	55.5	39.0	70.5	48.1
11.0	11.8	26.0	21.0	41.0	30.1	56.0	39.3	71.0	48.4
11.5	12.1	26.5	21.3	41.5	30.4	56.5	39.6	71.5	48.7
12.0	12.4	27.0	21.6	42.0	30.7	57.0	39.9	72.0	49.0
12.5	12.7	27.5	21.9	42.5	31.0	57.5	40.2	72.5	49.3
13.0	13.0	28.0	22.2	43.0	31.3	58.0	40.5	73.0	49.6
13.5	13.3	28.5	22.5	43.5	31.6	58.5	40.8	73.5	49.9
14.0	13.6	29.0	22.8	44.0	31.9	59.0	41.1	74.0	50.2
14.5	13.9	29.5	23.1	44.5	32.2	59.5	41.4	74.5	50.5
15.0	14.3	30.0	23.4	45.0	32.6	60.0	41.7	75.0	50.9
15.5	14.6	30.5	23.7	45.5	32.9	60.5	42.0	75.5	51.2

Reprinted, by permission, from The Cooper Institute, 2013, *Fitnessgram/Activitygram test administration manual,* updated 4th ed. (Champaign, IL: Human Kinetics), 102.

Appendix D

PACER Conversion Chart

Use this chart to convert scores from the 15-meter PACER to their 20-meter equivalents.

Level		Laps																		
1	15 m	1	2	3	4	5	6	7	8	9										
	20 m	1	2	2	3	4	5	5	6	7										
2	15 m	10	11	12	13	14	15	16	17	18	19									
	20 m	8	8	9	10	11	12	12	13	14	15									
3	15 m	20	21	22	23	24	25	26	27	28	29	30								
	20 m	15	16	17	18	18	19	20	21	22	22	23								
4	15 m	31	32	33	34	35	36	37	38	39	40	41	42							
	20 m	24	25	25	26	27	28	28	29	30	31	32	32							
5	15 m	43	44	45	46	47	48	49	50	51	52	53	54							
	20 m	33	34	35	35	36	37	38	38	39	40	41	41							
6	15 m	55	56	57	58	59	60	61	62	63	64	65	66	67						
	20 m	42	43	44	45	45	46	47	48	48	49	50	51	51						
7	15 m	68	69	70	71	72	73	74	75	76	77	78	79	80						
	20 m	52	53	54	55	55	56	57	58	58	59	60	61	61						
8	15 m	81	82	83	84	85	86	87	88	89	90	91	92	93	94					
	20 m	62	63	64	65	65	66	67	68	68	69	70	71	72	72					
9	15 m	95	96	97	98	99	100	101	102	103	104	105	106	107	108					
	20 m	73	74	75	75	76	77	78	78	79	80	81	82	82	83					
10	15 m	109	110	111	112	113	114	115	116	117	118	119	120	121	122	123				
	20 m	84	85	85	86	87	88	88	89	90	91	92	92	93	94	94				
11	15 m	124	125	126	127	128	129	130	131	132	133	134	135	136	137	138				
	20 m	95	96	97	98	98	99	100	101	102	102	103	104	105	105	106				
12	15 m	139	140	141	142	143	144	145	146	147	148	149	150	151	152	153	154			
	20 m	107	108	108	109	110	111	111	112	113	114	114	115	116	117	117	118			
13	15 m	155	156	157	158	159	160	161	162	163	164	165	166	167	168	169	170	171		
	20 m	119	120	121	121	122	123	124	124	125	126	127	128	128	129	130	130	131		
14	15 m	172	173	174	175	176	177	178	179	180	181	182	183	184	185	186	187	188		
	20 m	132	133	134	134	135	136	137	137	138	139	140	140	141	142	143	143	144		
15	15 m	189	190	191	192	193	194	195	196	197	198	199	200	201	202	203	204	205	206	
	20 m	145	146	147	147	148	149	149	150	151	152	152	153	154	154	155	156	156	157	
16	15 m	207	208	209	210	211	212	213	214	215	216	217	218	219	220	221	222	223	224	
	20 m	158	159	160	160	161	162	163	163	164	165	166	166	167	168	169	170	170	171	
17	15 m	225	226	227	228	229	230	231	232	233	234	235	236	237	238	239	240	241	242	243
	20 m	172	173	174	174	175	176	177	177	178	179	179	180	181	181	182	183	184	184	185
18	15 m	244	245	246	247	248	249	250	251	252	253	254	255	256	257	258	259	260	261	262
	20 m	186	187	188	188	189	190	190	191	192	193	193	194	195	196	197	197	198	199	200

Adapted, by permission, from The Cooper Institute, 2013, *Fitnessgram/Activitygram test administration manual,* updated 4th ed. (Champaign, IL: Human Kinetics), 98.

Appendix E

Data Forms

Data Entry Form, page 120

General Brockport Physical Fitness Test Form, page 122

Data Entry Form 👆

This form is a quick and easy way to record student information and develop an appropriate fitness test for students. All possible tests from the Brockport Physical Fitness Test are listed. Simply fill in data for the tests you have a student perform. You can then use this record when completing an individualized Brockport Physical Fitness Test form for analysis of each student's results.

Student name: _____ Gender: ___Male ___Female

ID No.: _____ IEP (yes or no): _____ Grade (if applicable): _____

Height (feet and inches): _____ Weight: _____ Month and year: _____

Classification (check one)

_____ general (without disability) _____ intellectual disability _____ visual disability

_____ spinal cord injury _____ cerebral palsy _____ congenital anomaly or amputation

Subclassification (check subclassification necessary for test item selection and for reporting results)

Visual (check one)

_____ runs with assistance

_____ runs without assistance

Spinal cord injury (check one)

_____ low-level quadriplegia (LLQ)

_____ paraplegia: wheelchair (PW)

_____ paraplegia: ambulatory (PA)

Cerebral Palsy (check one)

_____ C1 _____ C2U _____ C2L _____ C3 _____ C4 _____ C5 _____ C6 _____ C7 _____ C8

Congenital Anomaly (check one)

_____ one arm only _____ two arms only _____ one leg only _____ two legs only

_____ one arm, one leg (same side) _____ one arm, one leg (opposite sides)

Scores

I. Aerobic Functioning

_____ Mile: run/walk time (min/sec)

_____ 20 m (laps)

_____ 15 m (laps)

_____ TAMT (P/F)

II. Body composition

_____ Height (feet and inches)

_____ Weight (lbs.)

_____ Percent body fat (%)

_____ Triceps (mm)

_____ Triceps + subscapular (mm)

_____ Triceps + calf (mm)

_____ BMI

III. Musculoskeletal Functioning

A. Strength and Endurance

_____ Reverse curl (#)

_____ 40 m push/walk (P/F)

_____ Ramp test (feet)

_____ Push-ups (#)

_____ Seated push-ups (sec.)

_____ Pull-ups (#)

_____ Modified pull-ups (#)

_____ Dumbbell press (#)

_____ Bench press (#)

_____ Grip strength (kg)

_____ Isometric push-ups (sec.)

_____ Extended-arm hang (sec.)

_____ Flexed-arm hang (sec.)

_____ Curl-ups (#)

_____ Modified curl-ups (#)

B. Flexibility or Range of Motion

_____ Trunk lift (in.)

_____ Shoulder stretch, right (P/F)

_____ Shoulder stretch, left (P/F)

_____ Back-saver, right (in.)

_____ Back-saver, left (in.)

_____ Modified Thomas test (0-3)

_____ Modified Apley test (0-3)

_____ Target stretch test (0-2)

_____ Wrist extension, right

_____ Wrist extension, left

_____ Elbow extension, right

_____ Elbow extension, left

_____ Shoulder extension, right

_____ Shoulder extension, left

_____ Shoulder abduction, right

_____ Shoulder abduction, left

_____ Shoulder external rotation, right

_____ Shoulder external rotation, left

_____ Forearm supination, right

_____ Forearm supination, left

_____ Forearm pronation, right

_____ Forearm pronation, left

_____ Knee extension, right

_____ Knee extension, left

From J. Winnick and F. Short, 2014, _Brockport physical fitness test manual: A health-related assessment for youngsters with disabilities_ (Champaign, IL: Human Kinetics).

General Brockport Physical Fitness Test Form

Student name: _____ Gender: ___ Male ___ Female

Age (yr): _____ Height: _____ Weight: _____ Date: _____

Classification: _____ Subclassification: _____

This form identifies all test items on the Brockport Physical Fitness Test (BPFT). It can be used as a resource for developing a fitness test for a particular student, recording results, and matching results to fitness zones. The BPFT typically includes four to six test items: one for aerobic functioning, one for body composition, and at least two for musculoskeletal functioning. (The Target Stretch Test items are considered as a single test for this purpose.) It is recommended that an individualized specific test form for each student consisting only of the items taken on the test be subsequently developed for each student and be used for reporting results to students, parents, and guardians. The results may serve as a basis for developing individualized education programs (IEPs) for students.

Aerobic Functioning

Test item	Units of measure	Test scores	Adapted Fitness Zone (if applicable)	Healthy Fitness Zone
AEROBIC CAPACITY				
Mile run or walk	min/sec			
20 m (laps)	#			
15 m (laps)	#			
AEROBIC BEHAVIOR				
TAMT	P/F		None	

Body Composition

Test item	Units of measure	Test scores	Adapted Fitness Zone (if applicable)	Healthy Fitness Zone
Percent body fat	%		No AFZ for body composition	
Triceps	(mm)			
Triceps + subscapular	(mm)			
Triceps + calf	(mm)			
Body mass index				

Musculoskeletal Functioning

Test item	Units of measure	Test scores	Adapted Fitness Zone (if applicable)	Healthy Fitness Zone
STRENGTH AND ENDURANCE				
Reverse curl	#			
40 m push/walk	P/F			
Ramp test	feet			
Push-ups	#			
Seated push-ups	#			
Pull-ups	#			

Test Item	Units of measure	Test scores	Adapted Fitness Zone (if applicable)	Healthy Fitness Zone
Modified pull-ups	#			
Dumbbell press	#			
Bench press	#			
Grip strength	kg			
Isometric push-ups	sec.			
Extended-arm hang	sec.			
Flexed-arm hang	sec.			
Curl-ups	#			
Modified curl-ups	#			
FLEXIBILITY OR RANGE OF MOTION				
Trunk lift	#			
Shoulder stretch, right	P/F			
Shoulder stretch, left	P/F			
Back-saver sit-and-reach, right	in.			
Back-saver sit-and-reach, left	in.			
Modified Thomas test	0-3			
Modified Apley test	0-3			
Target stretch test	0-2			
Wrist extension, right	0-2			
Wrist extension, left	0-2			
Elbow extension, right	0-2			
Elbow extension, left	0-2			
Shoulder extension, right	0-2			
Shoulder extension, left	0-2			
Shoulder abduction, right	0-2			
Shoulder abduction, left	0-2			
Shoulder external rotation, right	0-2			
Shoulder external rotation, left	0-2			
Forearm supination, right	0-2			
Forearm supination, left	0-2			
Forearm pronation, right	0-2			
Forearm pronation, left	0-2			
Knee extension, right	0-2			
Knee extension, left	0-2			

Interpretation: _____

_____

Needs: _____

_____

From J. Winnick and F. Short, 2014, *Brockport physical fitness test manual: A health-related assessment for youngsters with disabilities* (Champaign, IL: Human Kinetics).

Appendix F

Frequently Asked Questions

What age levels and disabilities are encompassed by the Brockport Physical Fitness Test (BPFT)?

The BPFT is a health-related, criterion-referenced test developed to assess the physical fitness of youngsters aged 10 to 17 years with disability. It is specially designed for individuals with intellectual, visual, and orthopedic impairment, including cerebral palsy, spinal cord injury, congenital anomaly, and amputation. The test corresponds to health-related physical fitness tests geared to youth in the general population, particularly Fitnessgram.

Briefly, what are the typical steps in administering the BPFT?

The first step is to identify students to whom the BPFT will be administered. This process is enhanced by knowing the populations for whom the test is targeted. The next step is to identify the specific disability of an individual and to identify any subclassifications associated with the disability. For example, an individual with spinal cord injury may have a subclassification of "paraplegic—wheelchair." Similarly, an individual with visual impairment may run events either with or without assistance. Once classification and subclassification are known, recommended test items for the individual are selected using the test-item selection guide presented in the test manual. To assist with this step, a sample data entry form is presented in appendix E. Next, test items are administered, test results are recorded, and data are interpreted. The interpretation of results leads to the determination of fitness status and the identification of unique needs that provide the basis for physical fitness goals.

How does the BPFT relate to disabilities not specifically targeted by the BPFT?

Because it is not possible to create in advance a specific test for each disability, the BPFT suggests developing an appropriate test for students in nontargeted populations by personalizing test development according to the following steps:

- Identify and select health-related concerns of importance to the young person.
- Establish a desired personalized fitness profile with (or, as necessary, for) the individual.
- Select components and subcomponents of physical fitness to be assessed.
- Select test items to measure the selected fitness components and subcomponents.
- Select health-related, criterion-referenced standards and fitness zones by which to evaluate the individual's physical fitness.

Specific recommendations for following this process are presented in this manual.

What are the objectives of the BPFT?

The BPFT is designed to assess the criterion-referenced, health-related physical fitness of youngsters with disability. In essence, the BPFT provides information regarding the status of individuals in regard to their functional and physiological health. The test provides standards and fitness zones representing levels of performance that serve as bases for comparison or criteria for assessing performance. Standards for evaluating physical fitness are associated with three components of health-related fitness: aerobic functioning, body composition, and musculoskeletal functioning (including muscular strength, endurance, and flexibility or range of motion). The BPFT measures an individual's status in these categories by means of various test items. The fitness components are affected by habitual physical activity, and they relate to the individual's functional and physiological health. It is expected that appropriate physical activity will enhance test-item performance and the health-related components of fitness, which in turn will enhance health.

How does the BPFT relate to IEP (individualized education program) goals for physical education?

Physical education involves the development of physical fitness. The BPFT is an instrument designed to assess the health-related physical fitness of individuals with disability. Test results provide a basis for identifying unique physical fitness needs. In other words, if a young person does not meet a specific or general standard of physical fitness, or does not attain an adapted or Healthy Fitness Zone, a unique need is identified. Following analysis of unique needs, goals are developed that can be incorporated into the IEP of a student with disability. Thus the BPFT enables teachers to identify a student's present level of performance, set individualized objectives or benchmarks, and set goals reflecting health-related fitness based on recommended criteria (standards and fitness zones).

How is the BPFT coordinated with other tests of health-related fitness?

To the extent appropriate, individuals with disability should be assessed using inclusive tests, or tests designed for the general population. At times, however, such tests hold limited application for individuals with disability, and in such cases alternative assessment should be provided. The health-related concerns of youngsters with disability exceed, as well as differ from, those of youngsters in the general population. Specific disabilities may affect movement modes, movement abilities, and health-related physical fitness potential.

For example, an individual who is completely paralyzed in the lower extremities and uses a wheelchair is unable to demonstrate aerobic functioning by running a mile. For this individual, a different way must be found to demonstrate and assess aerobic functioning. Clearly, then, test items for measuring and assessing physical fitness may differ—that is, may require modification, deletion, or creation—for youngsters with disability because of the wide variation in need and ability. Finally, to the extent possible, the specific nature of a physical fitness test should be developed through personal association and interaction (personalization) with the students being tested.

It is possible for teachers to use only some of the test items in the BPFT for youngsters with disability. A teacher may administer a set number of test items from tests used for the general population, then use one or more items associated with the BPFT. Teachers in inclusive settings, for example, are encouraged to administer test items from their general test battery to youngsters both with and without disability, as appropriate. At times, however, either a test or a standard may need to be different for a young person with a disability. In these instances, the BPFT can serve as a reference for filling in gaps in a test battery for a particular individual. Teachers who use Fitnessgram as their general test battery will find it relatively easy to coordinate with the BPFT because of the similarity between test items and standards used in the two tests.

What standards and fitness zones are used in the BPFT, and how are they developed?

Once test items have been selected to measure components and subcomponents of physical fitness, standards and fitness zones are selected that serve as the criterion-referenced basis for assessing fitness with a health status orientation. In the BPFT, standards are designated as general or specific. A general standard is a target measure of physical fitness associated with the general population of youth or a standard that is not adjusted for effects of disability. Data for general standards in the BPFT are primarily based on two sources: Fitnessgram (for BPFT test items included in the Fitnessgram test) and Project Target (for BPFT test items not included in Fitnessgram). These standards are assumed to reflect levels of health-related physical fitness to be pursued that may be recommended at times for youngsters with disability as well as for the general population. General standards provide the basis for Healthy Fitness Zones (HFZs).

Specific standards are target measures of physical fitness associated with a defined category of persons or adjusted for the effects of disability. Specific standards are provided only for selected test items for specific target populations. They are determined by adjustments of data from general standards associated with Fitnessgram or derived from Project Target. They reflect at least minimally acceptable levels of health-related physical fitness adjusted for the effects of disability or a challenging and attainable performance level of physical fitness leading to health-related physical fitness (a Healthy Fitness Zone). Specific standards provide the basis for adapted fitness zones (AFZs).

In essence, standards and fitness zones are based on two health constructs: physiological health and functional health. The key is to determine the level of fitness test performance associated with positive health. For example, an acceptable level of aerobic capacity is one that reduces the risk of developing diseases and conditions in adulthood, including high blood pressure, coronary heart disease, obesity, diabetes, and some forms of cancer. Therefore, setting and meeting standards are crucial steps in personalizing health-related physical fitness. The values associated with standards are determined by means of a number of strategies, including logic, research, and expert opinion.

Appendix G

Teacher and Parent Overview

About the Brockport Physical Fitness Test (BPFT)

The BPFT is a health-related, criterion-referenced test developed to assess the physical fitness of youngsters aged 10 to 17 years with disability. It is designed especially for individuals with intellectual, visual, and orthopedic impairment, including cerebral palsy, spinal cord injury, congenital anomaly, and amputation. The test corresponds to health-related physical fitness tests geared to students in the general population. In fact, many of the test items are either the same as or similar to items used with students in the general population; others are adapted or added.

The BPFT includes three components of health-related fitness: aerobic functioning, body composition, and musculoskeletal functioning (including muscular strength, endurance, and flexibility or range of motion). The BPFT measures status in these component categories by means of various test items. The fitness components are affected by habitual physical activity, and they relate to an individual's functional and physiological health. It is expected that physical activity will enhance test-item performance and the health-related components of fitness, which in turn will enhance health.

The components of health-related fitness for each individual are generally assessed using four to six test items. Levels of performance are assessed by comparing test scores with standards and fitness zones in order to determine an individual's unique physical fitness needs.

Healthy Fitness Levels

The BPFT generally presents three levels of health-related physical fitness. Individuals at the lowest level need improvement in the specific area of fitness being measured. The second level, designated as an adapted fitness zone (AFZ), reflects at least a minimally acceptable level of health-related physical fitness adjusted for the effects of disability *or* an attainable performance level of physical fitness leading to a Healthy Fitness Zone. AFZs are based on specific standards, which are target measures for youngsters with a specific disability. The third level, designated as a Healthy Fitness Zone (HFZ), reflects an acceptable level of health-related fitness that is associated with the general population and is not adjusted for disability. HFZs are based on general standards, which are target measures for the general population.

The data for the general and specific standards and fitness zones used in the BPFT come from two sources: Fitnessgram (for test items in the BPFT that are also included in Fitnessgram) and Project Target (for BPFT test items not included in Fitnessgram). The Fitnessgram test (Cooper Institute, 2010) is a health-related physical fitness test designed primarily for youngsters without disability. Project Target was a federally funded prockject designed to provide data to support the development of specific and general standards and fitness zones for test items on the BPFT for youth with and without disability (Project Target, 1998). Figure G.1 distinguishes levels of physical fitness for the flexed-arm hang.

In cases where both specific and general standards are provided, it is generally recommended that performance levels be increased to reach HFZs. In cases where only general standards are provided (e.g., curl-ups), students are generally encouraged to perform to their best performance level. An exception occurs if a general standard has a single set value specified for a test item (e.g., trunk lift, shoulder stretch) and performance increases are not recommended and may even be discouraged.

If unique needs exist, then improvements in physical fitness performance are warranted, and individualized objectives may be set for the student. As appropriate, objectives should reflect progress toward AFZs and subsequently HFZs. It is recommended that objectives be consistent with those specified in an individualized education program (IEP).

Muscular Strength and Endurance

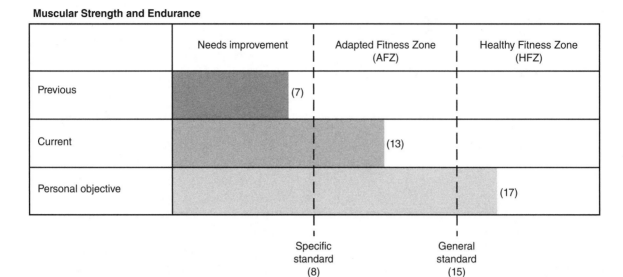

Figure G.1   Fitness zones for the flexed-arm hang (seconds).

Using the General Brockport Physical Fitness Test Form

The General Brockport Physical Fitness Test Form provides teachers with a way to communicate the health-related physical fitness status of each individual student with parents and students themselves. The form provides a place to track current and previous results for each test item and provides an opportunity to note goals and objectives based on results. On the report, teachers can indicate levels of performance (i.e., needs improvement, adapted fitness zones [AFZs], and Healthy Fitness Zones [HFZs]). Once this information is reviewed and analyzed, it may be used as a basis to set future objectives and goals. It is recommended that objectives and goals be added in the Interpretation and Needs sections as a part of the report and be consistent with the IEP of each youngster.

Standards and fitness zones in the report serve as the basis for determining unique needs for IEP development. A unique need and objective for an individual with a disability occurs when improvement is needed in order to attain a desired standard. If an AFZ is reached, then a unique need and an accompanying objective may be established to meet an HFZ unless contraindicated by the nature of the disability.

Glossary

adapted fitness zone (AFZ)—a fitness test score, or range of scores, deemed at least minimally acceptable or attainable for youngsters with a particular disability; it is delineated at the lower end by a specific standard and at the upper end by a general standard.

aerobic behavior—subcomponent of aerobic functioning that reflects the ability to sustain physical activity of a specific intensity for a particular duration.

aerobic capacity—subcomponent of aerobic functioning that reflects the maximal rate of oxygen consumption while exercising.

aerobic functioning—component of physical fitness that permits a person to sustain large-muscle, dynamic, moderate- to high-intensity activity for prolonged periods of time; includes the subcomponents of aerobic behavior and aerobic capacity.

body composition—component of health-related physical fitness involving the degree of body leanness or fatness.

body mass index (BMI)—index of the relationship between an individual's height and weight.

BMI = body weight (kilograms) / height² (meters)

BMI = body weight (pounds) × 704.5 / height² (inches)

components of physical fitness—categories or constructs that measure separate or unique aspects of fitness (e.g., the health-related components of fitness adopted for the Brockport Physical Fitness Test: aerobic functioning, body composition, and musculoskeletal functioning).

criterion-referenced standard—target measure of attainment against which a test score is judged (e.g., in the Brockport Physical Fitness Test); levels of attainment associated with physiological or functional health.

flexibility—subcomponent of musculoskeletal functioning that reflects the extent of movement possible in multiple joints while performing a functional task.

functional health—aspect of health that reflects an individual's physical capability, indexes of which include the ability to independently perform important tasks, independently sustain performance of those tasks, perform activities of daily living (ADLs), sustain physical activity, and participate in leisure activities.

general standard—a target measure of physical fitness appropriate for the general population of youngsters or a standard that is not adjusted for the effects of disability; general standards reflect fitness test scores associated with good health; at times general standards may be recommended for youngsters with disabilities as well as for the general population.

health—human condition with physical, social, and psychological dimensions, each characterized on a continuum with positive and negative poles . . . [wherein positive] health is associated with a capacity to enjoy life and to withstand challenges . . . [and thus] is not merely the absence of disease . . . [and wherein negative] health is associated with morbidity and, in the extreme, with premature mortality (Bouchard & Shephard, 1994); conceptualized in the Brockport Physical Fitness Test as having both functional and physiological aspects.

Healthy Fitness Zone (HFZ)—a fitness test score, or range of scores, deemed acceptable for youngsters in the general population; it is delineated at the lower end by a general standard and it may or may not have an upper boundary.

health-related physical fitness—(a) ability to perform and sustain daily activities and (b) demonstration of traits or capacities associated with low risk of premature development of diseases and conditions related to movement; fitness that involves components affected by habitual physical activity and related to health status.

individualized standard—desired level of attainment for an individual in an area of health status; established in consideration of his or her present level of performance and expectation for progress and not necessarily reflecting a health-related standard.

muscular endurance—subcomponent of musculoskeletal functioning that reflects the ability to repeatedly perform submaximal muscular contractions.

muscular strength—subcomponent of musculo-skeletal functioning that reflects the maximal amount of force that can be exerted.

musculoskeletal functioning—component of physical fitness combining muscular strength, muscular endurance, and flexibility or range of motion.

optional test item—alternative test item considered appropriate and acceptable for measuring a component of physical fitness.

physical activity—bodily movement produced by skeletal muscle resulting in a substantial increase over resting energy expenditure (Bouchard & Shephard, 1994).

physical fitness—set of attributes possessed or achieved that relate to one's ability to perform physical activity (Caspersen, Powell, & Christenson, 1985).

physiological health—aspect of health related to organic well-being, indexes of which include traits or capacities associated with well-being, absence of disease or condition, or low risk of developing a disease or condition.

profile—direction or broad goal for a health-related physical fitness program.

range of motion—subcomponent of musculo-skeletal functioning that reflects the extent of movement in a single joint.

recommended test item—test item considered appropriate and most acceptable for measuring physical fitness when other factors for selecting test items are equal.

specific standard—a target measure of physical fitness appropriate for a disability-specific category of persons or a standard that is adjusted for the effects of disability; specific standards reflect at least minimally acceptable levels of health-related physical fitness adjusted for the effects of disability or reflect attainable performance levels for youngsters with a disability that may lead to a general standard and health-related physical fitness; specific standards are provided only for selected test items for specific target populations.

References and Resources

American Association on Mental Retardation. (1992). *Mental retardation definition, classification, and systems of supports* (9th ed.). Washington, DC: Author.

Blair, S.N., Kohl, H.W., Gordon, N.F., & Paffenbarger, R.S., Jr. (1992). How much physical activity is good for health? *Annual Review of Public Health, 13,* 99–126.

Blair, S.N., Kohl, H.W., Paffenbarger, R.S., Jr., Clark, D.G., Cooper, K.H., & Gibbons, L.W. (1989). Physical fitness and all-cause mortality: A prospective study of healthy men and women. *Journal of the American Medical Association, 262,* 931–933.

Blair, S.N., Kohl, H.W., Paffenbarger, R.S., Jr., Clark, D.G., Cooper, K.H., & Gibbons, L.W. (1990). Physical fitness and all-cause mortality: A prospective study of healthy men. *Journal of the American Medical Association, 262,* 2395–2401.

Bouchard, C., & Shephard, R.J. (1994). Physical activity, fitness, and health: The model and key concepts. In C. Bouchard, R.J. Shephard, & T. Stephens (Eds.), *Physical activity, fitness, and health: International proceedings and consensus statement* (pp. 77–86). Champaign, IL: Human Kinetics.

Buell, C.E. (1983). *Physical education for blind children.* Springfield, IL: Charles C Thomas.

Caspersen, C.J., Powell, K.E., & Christenson, G.M. (1985). Physical activity, exercise, and physical fitness: Definitions and distinctions for health-related research. *Public Health Reports, 100,* 126–131.

Cerebral Palsy International Sports and Recreation Association. (1993). *CPISRA Handbook* (5th ed.). Heteren, Netherlands: Author.

Cole, T.M., & Tobis, J.S. (1990). Measurement of musculoskeletal function. In F.J. Kottke & J.F. Lehmann (Eds.), *Krusen's handbook of physical medicine and rehabilitation* (pp. 20–71). Philadelphia: Saunders.

Cooper Institute. (2007). *Fitnessgram & Activitygram test administration manual* (4th ed.). Champaign, IL: Human Kinetics.

Cooper Institute. (2010). *Fitnessgram & Activitygram test administration manual* (updated 4th ed.). Champaign, IL: Human Kinetics.

Cooper Institute. (2013). *FG 10: Addendum to the Fitnessgram & Activitygram test administration manual.* Dallas: Cooper Institute.

Cooper Institute for Aerobics Research. (1992). *The Prudential Fitnessgram test administration manual.* Dallas: Cooper Institute for Aerobics Research.

Cooper Institute for Aerobics Research. (1999). *Fitnessgram test administration manual.* Champaign, IL: Human Kinetics.

Cureton, K.J. (1994a). Aerobic capacity. In J.R. Morrow, H.B. Falls, & H.W. Kohl (Eds.), *The Prudential Fitnessgram technical reference manual* (pp. 33–55). Dallas: Cooper Institute for Aerobics Research.

Cureton, K.J. (1994b). Physical fitness and activity standards for youth. In R.R. Pate & R.C. Hohn (Eds.), *Health and fitness through physical education* (pp. 129–136). Champaign, IL: Human Kinetics.

Cureton, K.J., Sloniger, M.A., O'Bannon, J.P., Black, D.N. & McCormack, W.P. (1995). A generalized equation for prediction of $\dot{V}O_2$ peak from one-mile run/walk performance in youth. *Medicine and Science in Sports and Exercise, 27,* 445–451.

Cureton, K.J., & Warren, G.L. (1990). Criterion-referenced standards for youth health-related fitness tests: A tutorial. *Research Quarterly for Exercise and Sport, 61*(2), 7–19.

Eichstaedt, C., Polacek, J., Wang, P., & Dohrman, P. (1991). *Physical fitness and motor skill levels of individuals with mental retardation, ages 6–21.* Normal: Illinois State University.

Freedson, P.S. (1991). Electronic motion sensors and heart rate as measures of physical activity in children. *Journal of School Health, 61,* 220–223.

Freedson, P.S., & Melanson, E.L. (1996). Measuring physical activity. In D. Docherty (Ed.), *Measurement in pediatric exercise science* (pp. 261–283). Champaign, IL: Human Kinetics.

Government of Canada, Fitness and Amateur Sport. (1985). *Canada Fitness Award: Adapted for use by trainable mentally handicapped youth—A leader's manual* (Rev. ed.). Ottawa: Author.

Hayden, F.J. (1964). *Physical fitness for the mentally retarded.* Toronto: Metropolitan Toronto Association for Retarded Children.

Jansma, P., Decker, J., Ersing, W., McCubbin, J., & Combs, S. (1988). A fitness assessment system for individuals with severe mental retardation. *Adapted Physical Activity Quarterly, 5,* 223–232.

Johnson, R.E., & Lavay, B. (1989). Fitness testing for children with special needs: An alternative approach. *Journal of Physical Education, Recreation and Dance, 60*(6), 50–53.

Kosiak, M., & Kottke, F.J. (1990). Prevention and rehabilitation of ischemic ulcers. In F.J. Kottke & J.F. Lehmann (Eds.), *Krusen's handbook of physical medicine and rehabilitation* (pp. 976–987). Philadelphia: Saunders.

Leger, L.A., Mercier, D., Gadoury, C., & Lambert, J. (1988). The multistage 20-metre shuttle run test for aerobic fitness. *Journal of Sports Sciences, 6,* 93–101.

Lieberman, L.J., & Houston-Wilson, C. (2009). Strategies for inclusion: A handbook for physical educators. Champaign, IL: Human Kinetics.

Lohman, T.G. (1994). Body composition. In Cooper Institute for Aerobics Research, *The Prudential Fitnessgram technical reference manual* (pp. 57–72). Dallas: Cooper Institute for Aerobics Research.

McClain, J.J., Welk, G.J., Ihmels, M., & Schaben, J. (2006). Comparison of two versions of the PACER aerobic fitness test. *Journal of Physical Activity and Health, 3*(Suppl. 2), S476.

Pate, R.R. (1988). The evolving definition of fitness. *Quest, 40,* 174–178.

Plowman, S.A. (2008). Muscular strength, endurance, and flexibility assessments. In G.J. Welk & M.D. Meredith (Eds.), *Fitnessgram/Activitygram reference guide.* Dallas: Cooper Institute.

Plowman, S.A., & Corbin, C.B. (1994). Muscular strength, endurance, and flexibility. In J.R. Morrow, H.B. Falls, & H.W. Kohl (Eds.), *The Prudential Fitnessgram technical reference manual* (pp. 73–100). Dallas: Cooper Institute for Aerobics Research.

Project Target. (1998). In J.P. Winnick & F.X. Short, *Project Target: Criterion-referenced physical fitness standards for adolescents with disabilities, final report.* Project No. H023C30091-95 funded by the Office of Special Education and Rehabilitative Services, U.S. Department of Education. Brockport: State University of New York. (Eric Document Reproduction Service No. ED433627)

Project Target Advisory Committee. (1997, April 18–19). Meeting of the Project Target Advisory Committee, Brockport, NY. Notes from meeting.

U.S. Department of Health and Human Services. (1996). *Physical activity and health: A report of the Surgeon General.* Atlanta: U.S. Department of Health and Human Services, Centers for Disease Control and Prevention, National Center for Chronic Disease Prevention and Health Promotion.

U.S. Department of Health and Human Services. (2008). Physical activity guidelines for Americans. Office of Disease Prevention & Health Promotion. www.health.gov/paguidelines/guidelines/default.aspx#toc.

Waters, R.L. (1992). Energy expenditure. In J. Perry, *Gait analysis: Normal and pathological function* (pp. 443–487). Thorofare, NJ: Slack.

Welk, G.J., & Meredith, M.D. (Eds.). (2008). *Fitnessgram/Activitygram reference guide.* Dallas: Cooper Institute.

Welk, G., & Wood, K. (2000). Physical activity assessments in physical education: A practical review of instruments and their use in the curriculum. *Journal of Physical Education, Recreation and Dance, 71*(1), 30–40.

Winnick, J.P. (Ed.). (2011) *Adapted physical education and sport* (5th ed.). Champaign, IL: Human Kinetics.

Winnick, J.P., & Short, F.X. (1985). *Physical fitness testing of the disabled: Project UNIQUE.* Champaign, IL: Human Kinetics.

Winnick, J.P., & Short, F.X. (2005). Brockport Physical Fitness Test development. *Adapted Physical Activity Quarterly, 22*(4), 315–417.

Zhu, W., Plowman, S.A., & Park, Y. (2010). A primer-test centered equating method for setting cutoff scores. *Research Quarterly for Exercise and Sport, 81,* 400–409.

Index

Note: Page numbers followed by an italicized *t* or *f* indicate a table or figure will be found on those pages, respectively. Italicized *tt* or *ff* indicate multiple tables or figures will be found on those pages, respectively.

A

AAHPERD 1

activities of daily living (ADLs) 8

adapted fitness zones (AFZs)

    as a basis for fitness evaluation 11

    specific standards for 12

ADLs. *See* activities of daily living

aerobic behavior

    BPFT form 122

    described 9

    measure of 15

aerobic capacity. *See* $\dot{V}O_2$max

aerobic functioning

    BPFT form 122-123

    as a component of BPFT 9-11

    for the general population 31

    measure of 13-15

    one-mile run/walk 63-64

    PACER 58-59, 58*f*

    physical fitness data summary and profile 27*f*

    TAMT 59-62, 61*tt*

    test components of 18*f*

    test items and standards 25*t*

    test-item selection guide 30*t*, 38*t*

    for youngsters with cerebral palsy 37

    for youngsters with congenital anomalies 40*t*, 41

    for youngsters with intellectual disabilities 32

    for youngsters with spinal cord injuries 36

    for youngsters with visual impairments 34*t*

age considerations 56-57

alternative assessments 3, 4*t*, 101-102

alternative flexibility-testing apparatuses 110

American Alliance for Health, Physical Education, Recreation and Dance. *See* AAHPERD

American Association on Mental Retardation 3

American National Standards Institute (ANSI) 16-17

amputation. *See* youngsters with congenital anomalies

Apley test

    modified 88-89, 88*f*

    scoring 17

B

back-saver sit-and-reach

    Fitnessgram standards for boys 43*t*

    Fitnessgram standards for girls 44*t*

    to measure hamstring flexibility 89-90

    relationship to low-back pain 17

    resources for 108

back-saver sit-and-reach apparatus 109

barbells 69

bench press 69-70, 69*f*

bioelectrical impedance analysis (BIA) 68

Black, D.N. 13

blindness. *See* youngsters with visual impairments

BMI. *See* body mass index

body composition

    assessment of 15

    bioelectrical impedance analysis 68

    BPFT form 122

    as a component of BPFT 11

    described 9

    Fitnessgram conversion charts 115-116

    for the general population 31

    measurement of BMI 67

    measures of 15

    physical fitness data summary and profile 27*f*

    physical fitness parameters 33

    skinfold measurements 65-66, 65*f*

    subcomponents of 10

    test components of 19*f*

    test items and standards 25*t*

    test-item selection guide 30*t*, 38*t*

    for youngsters with cerebral palsy 37

body composition (*continued*)

for youngsters with congenital anomalies 40t, 41

for youngsters with spinal cord injuries 35t

for youngsters with visual impairments 34, 34t

body mass index (BMI)

assessment of 15

of boys with intellectual disability 45f

BPFT form 122

chart of values 106

computing 67

Fitnessgram standards for boys 43t

Fitnessgram standards for girls 44t

of girls with intellectual disability 46f

Brockport Physical Fitness Test (BPFT)

administering the test 23-24

fitness test items 11

frequently asked questions 125-127

index of test items 57

individualized nature of testing 2

overview of 1-2

physical fitness test form 122-123

profile statements 11, 18f-20f

recommendations for administering 55-56

target populations 3-6, 4t

teacher and parent overview of 129

test construction 2-3

test items by component 11

test items with available standards 25t

unique elements of 2

use of, with other tests 28

using the physical fitness test form 130

Buell, C.E. 14

C

calf skinfold measurements 65

Canada Fitness Award 18

cerebral palsy 14. *See* youngsters with cerebral palsy

Cerebral Palsy International Sports and Recreation Association (CPISRA) 4-5

children. *See the various youngsters categories*

Cole, T.M. 18

Combs, S. 101

congenital anomalies. *See* youngsters with congenital anomalies

Cooper Institute for Aerobics Research 17

CPISRA. *See* Cerebral Palsy International Sports and Recreation Association

criterion-referenced standards 1

Cureton, K.J. 13

curl-up measuring strips 108

curl-ups 108

Fitnessgram standards for boys 43t

Fitnessgram standards for girls 44t

modified 72

musculoskeletal functioning 71f-72f

D

Data Based Gymnasium 101

data collection for Project Target 18

data entry forms 120-121

data for standards 12

Decker, J. 101

desired profiles

for youngsters in the general population 30

for youngsters with cerebral palsy 37

for youngsters with congenital anomalies 39

for youngsters with intellectual disability 31

for youngsters with spinal cord injuries 35

for youngsters with visual impairments 33

disabilities effect on movement modes 9

Dohrman, P. 18

dominant grip strength 76-77, 76ff, 108

dumbbell press 73

dynamometers 76f

E

ecological task analysis 101

Eichstaedt, C. 18

elbow extension 94

electrical flow 68

electronic heart rate monitors 108

endurance tests

bench test 69-70

BPFT form 122

curl-ups 70-72, 71*f*-72*f*

dominant grip strength 76-77, 76*f*

extended-arm hang 74

flexed-arm hang 75, 130*f*

isometric push-ups 77-78, 77*f*

40-meter push/walk 82-83

modified pull-ups 79-80, 79*f*

pull-ups 78-80, 78*f*-79*f*

push-ups 80-81, 80*f*

reverse curl 84

seated push-ups 85

trunk lift 86

wheelchair ramp test 87

equipment

for the back-saver sit-and-reach 89-90

back-saver sit-and-reach apparatus 109

curl-up measuring strips 108

for curl-ups 70

for dominant grip strength 76

for the dumbbell press 73

electronic heart rate monitors 108

for the extended-arm hang 74

for the flexed-arm hang 75

for the isometric push-up 78

Jamar grip dynamometer 108

for measuring BMI 67

for the 40-meter push/walk 82

for the modified Thomas test 92

for the one-mile run/walk 63

for the PACER 58

PACER equipment 108

for pull-ups 79-80

push-up blocks 108

for push-ups 81

resources for 108

for the reverse curl 84

for seated push-ups 85

sit-and-reach apparatus 108

skinfold caliper 108

for skinfold measurements 66

for TAMT 60

for the target stretch test 95

for trunk lifts 86

for the wheelchair ramp test 87

equipment and construction steps

for back-saver sit-and-reach apparatus 109

for modified pull-up stand 113

for ramp 111-112

Ersing, W. 101

extended-arm hang 74

F

fat levels in the body 15, 65

fitness forms 130*f*

Fitnessgram

AAHPERD adoption of 1

BMI standards for boys 43*t*

BMI standards for girls 44*t*

body composition conversion charts 115-116

described 129

health-related concerns 10

overview of 1

$\dot{V}O_2$max standards for boys 43*t*

$\dot{V}O_2$max standards for girls 44*t*

fitness zones 17-18, 19*f*-22*f*

flexed-arm hang 75, 130*f*

flexibility tests 17

alternative apparatuses 110

back-saver sit-and-reach 89-90, 89*f*

BPFT form 123

modified Apley test 88-89

modified Thomas test 92-93, 93*f*

shoulder stretch 91

target stretch test 94-100, 96*t*, 97*f*-99*f*

test components for 22*f*

valid measures of 17

flow, electrical 68

forearm pronation 95

forearm supination 95

forms

Brockport physical fitness test form 122-123

data entry 120-121

physical fitness data summary and profile 27*f*

physical fitness profile sheet 26*f*

for target stretch tests 97*f*-99*f*

frequently asked questions 125-127
functional health 7-8

G

general population. *See* youngsters in the general population
goniometer 95, 96*t*
Good, Pat 59
Gopher Sport 108
grip dynamometer 76*f*

H

hamstring muscles 89-90
Hayden, F.J. 18
health
    definition of 7
    and musculoskeletal functioning 15
    relationships between activity and fitness 8*t*
health-related concerns
    for youngsters in the general population 30, 30*t*
    for youngsters with cerebral palsy 37
    for youngsters with congenital anomalies 39
    for youngsters with intellectual disability 31
    for youngsters with spinal cord injuries 35
    for youngsters with visual impairments 33
health-related physical fitness, definition of 9
healthy fitness levels 129-130, 130*f*
Healthy Fitness Zones (HFZs)
    as a basis for fitness evaluation 11
    specific standards for 12
    standards for boys 43*t*
    standards for girls 44*t*
heart rate monitors 82
heart rate values 61*t*
hip flexor muscles 92
Human Kinetics 108

I

I CAN 101
individualized education programs (IEPs)
    adapting fitness standards 24
    developing 28

individualized standards 12
intellectual disability. *See* youngsters with intellectual disability
isometric push-up 77-78, 77*f*, 103*ft*

J

Jamar grip dynamometer 32*t*-33*t*, 76, 108
Jansma, P. 101
Johnson, R.E. 69
joints, movement extent in 94

K

knee extension 95

L

Lange skinfold caliper 66*f*
Lavay, B. 69
low-level quadriplegia (LLQ) 4

M

McCormack, W.P. 13
McCubbin, J. 101
mental retardation. *See* youngsters with intellectual disability
40-meter push/walk 16, 82-83, 82*f*-83*f*
mile run/walk formula 13
motivation for the PACER test 58
musculoskeletal functioning
    back-saver sit-and-reach 90
    bench press 69-70, 69*f*
    BPFT form 122
    as a component of BPFT 11
    as a component of fitness 9
    curl-ups 70-72, 71*f*-72*f*
    dominant grip strength 76-77, 76*ff*
    dumbbell press 73
    extended-arm hang 74
    flexed-arm hang 75, 130*f*
    for the general population 31
    isometric push-up 77-78, 77*f*
    measures of 15-17
    40-meter push/walk 82-83, 82*f*-83*f*
    modified Apley test 88-89, 88*f*

modified Thomas test 92-93, 93*f*

physical fitness data summary and profile 27*f*

physical fitness parameters 33

pull-ups 78-80, 78*f*-79*f*

push-ups 80-81, 80*f*

reverse curl 84

seated push-up 85

shoulder stretch 91

subcomponents of 10

target stretch test 94

test items and standards 25*t*

test-item selection guide 30*t*, 38*t*

trunk lifts 86

wheelchair ramp test 87

of youngsters with cerebral palsy 37

of youngsters with congenital anomalies 40*t*, 41

of youngsters with spinal cord injuries 35*t*, 36

of youngsters with visual impairments 34*t*

N

negative health 7

O

O'Bannon, J.P. 13

obesity 15

one-mile run/walk 63-64

P

PACER 108

aerobic functioning 58-59, 58*f*

for boys with intellectual disability 45*f*

conversion chart 117

Fitnessgram standards for boys 43*t*

Fitnessgram standards for girls 44*t*

for girls with intellectual disabilities 46*t*

lap standards 14

paraplegia 4, 5*t*, 16

Patterson Medical 108

personalized approach to testing 2, 11

personalized profile 10

physical activity

described 7

measurement of 102, 103*ft*

relationships between health, physical fitness, and 8*t*

physical fitness

Brockport test form 122-123

components of 10, 30

criterion-referenced test of 1

health-related 9

health-related concerns 9-10

parameters for testing 23-24

personalized approach to 9-10

relationships between activity and health 8*t*

sample profile sheet 26*f*

testing and evaluating 23-24, 25*t*, 26*f*-27*f*

physical fitness parameters

for youngsters in the general population 30-31, 30*t*

for youngsters with congenital anomalies 39-41, 40*t*, 42*t*

for youngsters with intellectual disability 31-33, 32*t*

for youngsters with spinal cord injuries 35-36, 35*t*

physiological health 7

Polacek, J. 18

positive health 7

profiles. *See* desired profiles

profile statements 10

Project MOBILITEE 101

Project Target

about 129

data collected for 18

described 12

funding for 1

Project Target Advisory Committee 17-18

Project Transition assessment system 101

project UNIQUE 18

Prudential Fitnessgram 1

pull-ups 78-80, 78*f*-79*f*

push-up, isometric 77-78, 77*f*

push-up blocks 108

push-ups 80-81, 80*f*

Q

quadriplegia 5*t*

R

range of motion tests 17
    back-saver sit-and-reach 89-90, 89*f*
    BPFT form 123
    functional 17
    modifications for the dumbbell press 73
    modified Apley test 88-89
    modified Thomas test 92-93, 93*f*
    seated push-up modification 85
    shoulder stretch 91
    target stretch test 96*t*, 97*f*-99*f*
ratings of perceived exertion 83
recommended test item 24
reliability of test items 2
reverse curl 16, 84
rubric for isometric push-up 103*f*

S

safety guidelines and precautions 56
sample task analysis 103*f*
scoring and trials
    for the back-saver sit-and-reach 89-90
    for the bench press 70
    for curl-ups 70-71
    for dominant grip strength 77
    for the dumbbell press 73
    for the extended-arm hang 74
    for the flexed-arm hang 75
    for the isometric push-up 78
    for measuring BMI 67
    for the 40-meter push/walk 82
    for the modified Apley test 88
    for the modified Thomas test 92
    for the one-mile run/walk 63
    for the PACER 58
    for pull-ups 79
    for push-ups 81
    for the reverse curl 84
    for seated push-ups 85
    for the shoulder stretch 91
    for skinfold measurements 66
    for TAMT 60
    for trunk lifts 86
    using a goniometer 95
    for the wheelchair ramp test 87
seated push-up 16, 85, 108
Short, F.X. 2, 11, 13
shoulder abduction 94
shoulder extension 94
shoulder external rotation 94
shoulder stretch 91
sit-and-reach apparatus 108
skinfold measurements 65-66, 65*f*, 108
    body composition conversion charts 115-116
skinfold sites 15
Sloniger, M.A. 13
specific standards 12
spinal cord injuries 61-62. *See* youngsters with spinal cord injuries
standards and fitness zones
    for adapted fitness zones 12
    aerobic capacity 14
    basis for 12-13
    criterion-referenced 1
    data for 12
    general 12
    for the general population 30-31
    individualized 12
    for the 40-meter push/walk 16
    for modified tests 38-39
    for musculoskeletal functioning 16
    for the seated push-up 16
    sources of 17-18, 19*f*-22*f*
    for the wheelchair ramp test 16-17
    for youngsters with cerebral palsy 37
    for youngsters with congenital anomalies 41
    for youngsters with intellectual disabilities 32
    for youngsters with spinal cord injuries 36
    for youngsters with visual impairments 33-34, 34*t*
subscapular skinfold measurements 65

T

target aerobic movement test (TAMT)

about 108

BPFT form 122

to measure aerobic behavior 15

scoring and trials 60

target heart rate 59-60

test modifications for 60-61, 61t

target stretch test (TST)

for flexibility or range of motion 94-100, 96t, 97f-99f

goniometric values associated with 96t

as a subject measurement of movement 17

test administration suggestions

for the back-saver sit-and-reach 90

for bench press 70

for curl-ups 70-71

for dominant grip strength 77

for dumbbell press 73

for extended-arm hang 74

for the flexed-arm hang 75

for the isometric push-up 78

for the 40-meter push/walk 83

for the modified Apley test 89

for the modified Thomas test 93

for the one-mile run/walk 63-64

for PACER 59

for pull-ups 79

for push-ups 81

for the reverse curl 84

for seated push-ups 85

for the shoulder stretch 91

for skinfold measurements 66

for TAMT 61-62

for target stretch tests 100

for trunk lifts 86

for the wheelchair ramp test 87

test construction 2-3

test items, index of 57

test-item selection guides 24

for youngsters with cerebral palsy 38t

for youngsters with congenital anomalies 40t

for youngsters with intellectual disabilities 32

for youngsters with spinal cord injuries 35t

for youngsters with visual impairments 34t

test modifications

for the back-saver sit-and-reach 90

for the bench press 70

for curl-ups 70-71

for the dumbbell press 73

for the extended-arm hang 74

for measuring BMI 67

for the 40-meter push/walk 82

for the modified Thomas test 92

for the one-mile run/walk 63

for the PACER 58-59, 58f

for pull-ups 79

for push-ups 81

for the reverse curl 84

for seated push-ups 85

for the shoulder stretch 91

for skinfold measurements 66

for TAMT 60-61, 61t

for target stretch tests 100

for trunk lifts 86

for the wheelchair ramp test 87

Thomas test 17, 92-93, 93f

Tobis, J.S. 18

traumatic spinal cord injury 5

triceps skinfold measurements 65, 115-116

trunk and abdominal functioning 21f

trunk lift

Fitnessgram standards for boys 43t

Fitnessgram standards for girls 44t

trunk lifts 86

U

unilateral test items 16

upper-body flexibility 91

U.S. Association of Blind Athletes (USABA) 4

U.S. Chemical 108

V

validity of test items 2

visual impairments. *See* youngsters with visual impairments

$\dot{V}O_2$max
  adjustment of standards 14
  and aerobic functioning 9
  equation for estimating 13-15
  Fitnessgram standards for boys 43t
  Fitnessgram standards for girls 44t
  standards in the BPFT 14
  in youngsters with cerebral palsy 14

W
walking speed in adults 16
Wang, P. 18
wheelchair exercises
  dumbbell press 73
  ramp test 87
  reverse curls 84
  seated push-up 85
wheelchair ramp test, standards for 16-17
Winnick, J.P. 2, 11, 13, 101
wrist extension 94

Y
youngsters in the general population
  physical fitness parameters for 30-31, 30t
  test-item selection guide for 30t
youngsters with cerebral palsy
  classification system for 4-6

  estimating $\dot{V}O_2$max in 14
  fitness zone table for 51f, 52t
  physical parameters for 37-39, 38t
youngsters with congenital anomalies
  fitness zone table for 53f-54f
  physical fitness parameters for 39-41, 40t
  subclassification of 8
  test-item selection guide for 40t
youngsters with intellectual disabilities
  assessment of physical fitness 3, 4t
  components of physical fitness for 31, 32t
  definition of intellectual disability 3
  physical fitness parameters for 31-33
  standards for 14
  test-item selection guide for 32t
  test modifications for PACER 58
  test modifications for trunk lifts 86
youngsters with spinal cord injuries
  BPFT test items for 4, 5t
  fitness zone table for 49t, 50f
youngsters with visual impairments
  adjusting BPFT for 28
  fitness zone table for 47t, 48f
  limitations and needs of 4, 4t
  physical fitness parameters for 33-34, 34t
  test modifications for PACER 58

Contributors

Central Staff at the College at Brockport, State University of New York

Project director: Joseph P. Winnick

Project coordinator: Francis X. Short (1994–1998)

George Lawther (1993–1994)

Graduate assistants

Kevin Biata

Mary Powers

Rob Korzeniewski

Kevin Wexler

Lori Erickson

Office of Special Education and Rehabilitative Services, Washington, DC

Project Officer: Melville Appell

Project Target Advisory Committee and Panel of Experts

Kirk J. Cureton, PhD, University of Georgia

Harold W. Kohl, PhD, Baylor Sports Medicine Institute

Kenneth Richter, DO, medical director, U.S. Cerebral Palsy Athletic Association

James H. Rimmer, PhD, Northern Illinois University

Margaret Jo Safrit, PhD, American University

Roy J. Shephard, MD, PhD, DPE, University of Toronto (retired)

Julian U. Stein, EdD, George Mason University (retired)

Consultants

Patrick DiRocco, University of Wisconsin at La Crosse

Bo Fernhall, George Washington University

Georgia Frey, Texas Tech University

Timothy G. Lohman, University of Arizona

Jeffrey McCubbin, Oregon State University

Paul Surburg, Indiana University

Field Testers

Dianne Agostinelli

Matthew Beaty

Ron Berman

Kevin Biata

Kelly Bissell

Joel Blakeman

Karenne Bloomgarden

Ed Carll

Tim Baird

Mary Coe

Fiona Connor-Kuntz

Tim Coyle

Carol Brun Del Re

Kelda DePrez

Ben Drake

Kathryn Efthimiades

Bo Fernhall

Deborah Follis

Jean Friedel

Ellen Gill

Gerard Gonsalves

Victoria Gross

Terri Hansen

David Haveman

Wendy Kohler

Shelly Kron

Lauren Lieberman

Tosha Litwinski

Laura Mauer

Nancy McNulty

Alayne Miller

Stephen O'Hanlon

Travis Phillips

Kenneth Pitetti

Elizabeth Pitts

Mary Powers

Dana Rieger

James Rimmer

Maria Rodriguez

Amy Roska

Laura Scala

David Seefeldt

Michelle Shea

Steve Skaggs

Louis Stadler

Eric Stern

Nancy Stubbs

Mary Szekely

Cindy Thomas

Lori Volding

Matthew Vukovich

Mary Walsh

Kevin Wexler

Stephanie White

Matthew Wilkins

Melissa Zurlo

Other Contributors

Val Benzing, Brockport, NY

Jean Berry, Brockport, NY

Dixie Butler, Brockport, NY

Michael Coriale, Brockport, NY

Mel Eisenback, New York, NY

Robert Ellis, Brockport, NY

Arnie Epstein, New York, NY

Sister Seraphine Herbst, Rochester, NY

Jack Hogan, Brockport, NY

Sam Hughes, Houston Independent School District, TX

Pat Johnson, Brockport, NY

Bob Jones, Brockport, NY

Brian Jones, Brockport, NY

Richard Kingdon, Brockport, NY

Robert Lewis, New York, NY

Pam Maryjanowski, Brockport, NY

Gregory Packard, Brockport, NY

Fred Parker, Brockport, NY

Paul Ponchillia, Western Michigan University

Jack Purificato, Brockport, NY

Joseph Setek, Brockport, NY

Pam Siedlecki, Brockport, NY

William Straub, Ithaca, NY

Wendy Wheeler, Brockport, NY

Testing Projects

Brockport Central School District Brockport, NY

Empire State Games for the Physically Challenged, Brockport, NY

George Washington University Project, Washington, DC

Houston Independent School District, Houston, TX

Michigan State School for the Blind, Lansing, MI

New York City Public Schools

Northern Illinois University Project, DeKalb, IL

Oregon State University, Corvallis, OR

Paralympic Games, Atlanta, GA

School of the Holy Childhood, Rochester, NY

Western Michigan University, Kalamazoo, MI

About the Authors

Joseph P. Winnick, EdD, is a distinguished service professor of physical education and sport at the College at Brockport, State University of New York. He received master's and doctoral degrees from Temple University. Dr. Winnick developed and implemented America's first master's degree professional preparation program in adapted physical education at Brockport in 1968 and since that time has secured funds from the U.S. Department of Education to support the program. He continues to be involved in research related to the physical fitness of persons with disabilities. Dr. Winnick has received the G. Lawrence Rarick Research Award and the Hollis Fait Scholarly Contribution Award and is a three-time recipient of the Amazing Person Award from the New York Association for SHAPE America—formerly known as the American Alliance for Health, Physical Education, Recreation and Dance (AAHPERD). He has also received a Career Achievement Award from the College at Brockport and is a fellow in the Research Consortium of AAHPERD.

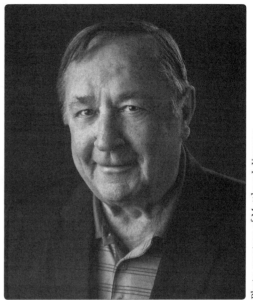

Photo courtesy of Matthew J. Yeoman.

Francis X. Short, PED, is professor and dean of the School of Health and Human Performance at the College at Brockport, State University of New York. Dr. Short has been involved with adapted physical education programs for over 40 years. He has coauthored numerous journal articles related to physical fitness and youngsters with disabilities. He also has authored and coauthored books and chapters related to adapted physical education. Dr. Short has served as project coordinator for three federally funded research projects pertaining to physical fitness and youngsters with disabilities and is a recipient of the G. Lawrence Rarick Research Award. He is a member of SHAPE America—formerly known as the American Alliance for Health, Physical Education, Recreation and Dance (AAHPERD)—and the National Consortium for Physical Education and Recreation for Individuals with Disabilities.

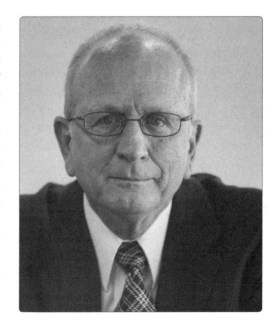

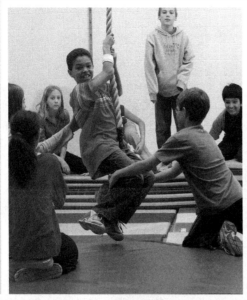
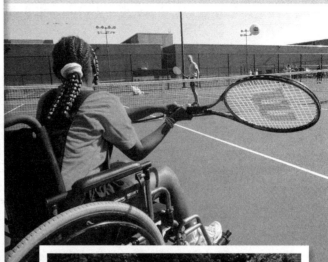
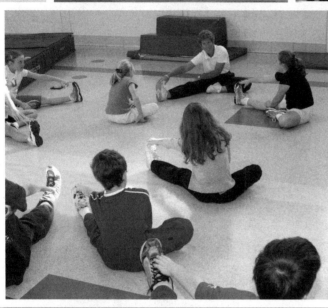
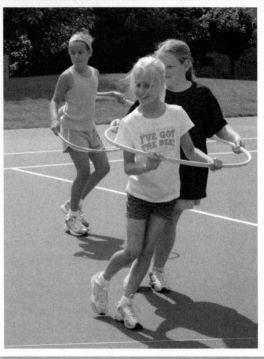
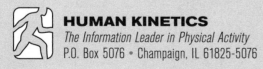